DENTAL MORPHOLOGY
an illustrated guide

Geoffrey C. van Beek BDS (Brist)

With a Foreword by
D. J. Anderson BDS MSc PhD LDS RCS
Professor of Oral Biology in the University of Bristol

Second edition

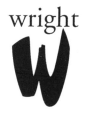

wright

WRIGHT
An imprint of Elsevier Limited

First published 1975
Second edition 1983
Reprinted 1986, 1991, 1992 (twice), 1993, 1995, 1996, 1997, 1999, 2000, 2001, 2002, 2003, 2005

ISBN 0 7236 0666 8

British Library Cataloguing in Publication Data
Van Beek, G. C.
  Dental morphology – 2nd ed.
  1. Teeth
  I. Title
  611.'314   QM331

Library of Congress Catalog Card Number
82-50780

Notice
Medical knowledge is constantly changing. Standard safety precautions must be followed, but as new research and clinical experience broaden our knowledge, changes in treatment and drug therapy may become necessary or appropriate. Readers are advised to check the most current product information provided by the manufacturer of each drug to be administered to verify the recommended dose, the method and duration of administration, and contraindications. It is the responsibility of the practitioner, relying on experience and knowledge of the patient, to determine dosages and the best treatment for each individual patient. Neither the Publisher nor the editors/contributor assumes any liability for any injury and/or damage to persons or property arising from this publication.

The Publisher

your source for books,
journals and multimedia
in the health sciences
www.elsevierhealth.com

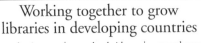
Working together to grow
libraries in developing countries

www.elsevier.com | www.bookaid.org | www.sabre.org

ELSEVIER   BOOK AID International   Sabre Foundation

The
Publisher's
policy is to use
paper manufactured
from sustainable forests

Typeset by Scribe Design, Gillingham, Kent
Printed and bound in Great Britain by MPG Books Ltd, Bodmin, Cornwall

Preface

The aim of this book is to present to the student the salient features of dental morphology within a new and simplified format. A technique of draughtmanship hitherto confined to technical drawing (*see* 'Explanation of Illustrative Technique') and a new and different lay-out of the text are employed to this end. It has been the author's intention to avoid expanding into the laborious, and perhaps unnecessarily lengthy descriptions which are to be found in certain other textbooks on this subject. This volume has been designed to be as convenient for reference as possible, and it is hoped that this will make it of particular assistance to dental students revising before, for example, an anatomy viva.

The illustrations consist entirely of line drawings. Photographs have been avoided for two reasons: first, that a photograph can only depict any one particular tooth, which could prove misleading. The author has drawn an average from a consideration of as many examples as possible. He has used every tooth from his collection of over one thousand fully-catalogued extracted teeth. To the best of the author's knowledge, most of the teeth are British, collected mainly from the south-west of England. All the examples of a particular tooth were set up in a line on long strips of wax, enabling an average tooth of each type to be judged by the artistic eye and drawn within the limits of the dimensions shown in the tables at the back of this book. Secondly, a photograph in reproduction tends to lose definition and detail, which may also tend to mislead. The right tooth of every pair has been shaded, the left is a simple line drawing. This will assist any student who may wish to copy drawings into his own notes. Schematic line drawings of the permanent teeth have also been included as a guide to wax carving for the student and the dental technician.

The design of the text allows for easy reference/swotting. A chronological table of tooth development is followed by a short general description. Unique to this book is the ordered list of principal identifying features, with the most helpful of these in italic type. A 'Variations' section has been included. The student should find it easier to refer to a separate section rather than be compelled to read through the entire description of a tooth in order to extract the necessary information. The present volume, however, is *not* designed to be fully comprehensive as regards racial or pathological variations, nor is it the author's intention to embark on a safari through the tiger-country of 'occlusion'! Changes in shape due to various wear patterns have only been mentioned where the author has considered it important in the identification of a tooth. It is felt that these subjects extend beyond the intended scope of this small book and they have been omitted accordingly. This is, after all, designed simply to be a tooth 'Identikit'. Cross-references have been added at the end of each tooth description with the intention of encouraging comparison with other teeth where indicated.

The deciduous dentition, which is no less important for the purposes of study than the permanent dentition, is fully described in the first section. It is hoped that the student will find this section of particular use, as the deciduous teeth are frequently summarily dismissed in other textbooks. A description of the permanent dentition is dealt with in the second section. A new, third section, 'Endodontic Anatomy' appears in this edition adding another dimension by describing the internal as well as the external morphology of the teeth, the importance of which extends into the clinical stage of the student's career in the field of endodontics. The final section contains some useful tables concerning the chronology of tooth development, and average tooth dimensions, as well as a glossary. A short bibliography has also been included.

All constructive criticism contributed since the publication of the first English and Dutch editions, has been considered in the revision of this second English edition, whilst still adhering as rigidly as possible to the original concept of producing a compact manual at a price which the undergraduate student, for whom this book is primarily intended, can easily afford. It is, however, evident, that each university has developed its own system of teaching, and that there exist, in some cases, quite remarkable differences of opinion between them on this subject. Controversy has therefore been avoided wherever possible in order to prevent unnecessary confusion, and blank spaces have been provided throughout the book for the student's own notes, should his lectures not be fully in agreement with a chapter. This has been done to allow this book to harmonize with most dental anatomy teaching courses.

The author wishes to acknowledge his gratitude to those teachers of the University of Bristol Medical and Dental Schools who helped to make this book possible, especially Professor D. J. Anderson, Dr R. J. Andlaw, and Professor G. Charlton.

Finally, credit must be given to Miss H. J. Deighton and Miss L. Dickinson for the typescript of the second edition.

Contents

Foreword

by Professor D. J. Anderson BDS MSc PhD LDS RCS
Professor of Oral Biology in the University of Bristol

In the Foreword to the first edition of this book, produced by Geoffrey Downer when he was a student, I said that it deserved to become popular. Since then the student has graduated; he has undergone a metamorphosis to become Geoffrey van Beek, he is a successful dental practitioner in Holland and following an edition in Dutch, we are now presented with the second English edition. So the expectations aroused by the first edition were fully justified.

The author has set out in the Preface the changes he has introduced in the format and content since the first edition appeared and his judgement in making these revisions and additions is obviously sound. As before, the presentation and the drawings are admirable, with the new section on Endodontic Anatomy providing very useful additional information.

It was remarkable that a student beset by the demands of the dental clinical curriculum was able to write a book which in its day was the only one devoted to dental morphology. It still retains this distinction and it is hardly less remarkable that a busy dental practitioner has sustained an interest and involvement in this subject to enable him within the space of a few years to revise and upgrade his first effort and publish it in two languages. I hope that all his teachers are proud of their pupil; this one most certainly is.

Explanation of Illustrative Technique

The illustrations in this book have been drawn in such a way as to relate the mesial, distal, buccal and lingual surfaces directly to the occlusal aspect in the hope of simplifying the visualization of the teeth as three-dimensional objects. This method of drawing is used by engineering draughtsmen to illustrate complicated machine parts, except that with machine parts one refers to 'Elevation A' and not 'Buccal aspect'. It is known technically as 'Third Angle Projection'.

Imagine that you have built a small glass cube around a tooth whose occlusal surface is uppermost (*Fig. 1*). Now, when viewing the distal, mesial, buccal and

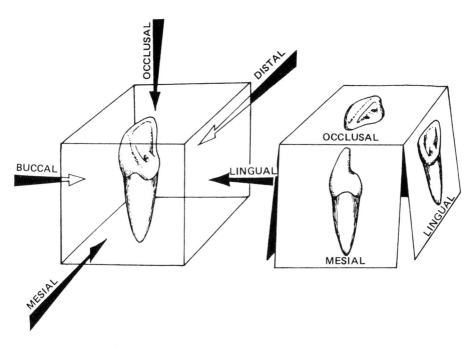

Fig. 1.   Fig. 2.

lingual surfaces of the tooth through the adjacent glass sides, imagine that the images you see can be transfixed onto the glass sides (*Fig. 2*) and hinged upwards into the same plane as the occlusal surface. You now have a third angle projection of the tooth (*Fig. 3*).

1

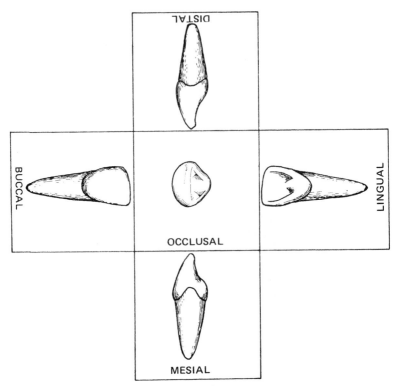

Fig. 3.

Terms of Reference in Tooth Identification

In the definition of a tooth, five things must be considered:
1. Is it a deciduous or a permanent tooth?
2. Is it an incisor, a canine, a premolar or a molar?
3. Is it a maxillary or a mandibular tooth?
4. If it is an incisor is it central or lateral?
   If it is a premolar, is it first or second?
   If it is a molar, is it first, second or third?
5. Does it come from the right or left side of the jaw?

It is important to remember that the terms 'right' or 'left' must always refer to the patient's right or left, not the dentist's.

The student is referred to the glossary for an explanation of the meaning of descriptive dental terms employed here and throughout the book.

In order that the notation of a tooth may be rendered speedier and simpler, a form of dental shorthand is employed. The following describes the most widely used system, namely the FDI (Fédération Dentaire Internationale) two-digit system:

Teeth are referred to by number, beginning at the vertical midline of the jaws, between the central incisors (*Fig. 4*).

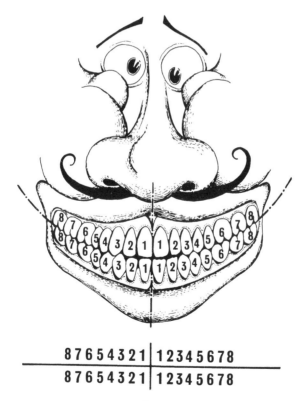

8 7 6 5 4 3 2 1	1 2 3 4 5 6 7 8
8 7 6 5 4 3 2 1	1 2 3 4 5 6 7 8

Fig. 4.

In the permanent dentition, therefore, the teeth are numbered 1 to 8 respectively from the central incisor to the third molar, and in the deciduous dentition 1 to 5 respectively from the central incisor to the second molar.

A single digit is, however, insufficient to describe a tooth fully in shorthand and extra information is necessary in order to determine if the tooth in question comes from the right or left side of the jaw, if it is a maxillary or mandibular tooth, or if it is a deciduous or permanent tooth. All this information is given by an extra digit placed in front of the number of the tooth, and refers to one of the four quadrants of either the permanent or the deciduous dentition (*Fig. 5*). The quadrant numbers are allocated as follows, beginning with the permanent dentition:

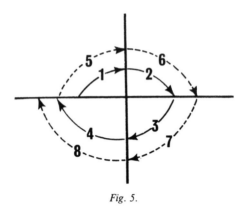

Fig. 5.

Permanent Dentition

1 Maxillary right
2 Maxillary left
3 Mandibular left
4 Mandibular right

The numerical order of the quadrants is clockwise and it continues for one more cycle in the same direction for the deciduous dentition as follows:

Deciduous Dentition

5 Maxillary right
6 Maxillary left
7 Mandibular left
8 Mandibular right

Some examples:

Maxillary right permanent central incisor	11
Maxillary left deciduous second molar	65
Maxillary left permanent lateral incisor	22
Mandibular right permanent second molar	47
Mandibular right deciduous canine	83

4

An alternative system with which the student should familiarize himself is the Zsigmond System. This older form of dental shorthand is still used in many dental schools and practices, especially in Great Britain and Ireland. Its construction is, however, somewhat cumbersome for microprocessor data storage, whereas that of the FDI system is not, and many dentists are of the opinion that as a result, the Zsigmond System can be regarded as yet another endangered species threatened by modern technology!

Teeth are referred to by number, 1–8, in the permanent dentition, and by letter A–E in the deciduous dentition. 1 or A is the first tooth from the midline, 2 or B the second, and so on.

The jaws are divided into quadrants by an imaginary cross, with a vertical line separating the right and left halves at the midline between the central incisors, and a horizontal line separating the lower and upper jaws (*Fig. 4*). In order to record any particular tooth, its number or letter is partially framed by means of an L-shaped symbol formed by a line at the appropriate side, to indicate left or right, and above or below to indicate maxillary or mandibular provenance.

Some examples:

Maxillary right permanent central incisor	1⌋
Maxillary left deciduous central incisor	⌊A
Mandibular left deciduous first molar	⌈D
Mandibular right second premolar	5⌉
Maxillary right permanent third molar	8⌋
Maxillary left deciduous canine	⌈C

FDI System (Fédération Dentaire Internationale)

Permanent Dentition

Maxillary right   Maxillary left

18	17	16	15	14	13	12	11	21	22	23	24	25	26	27	28
48	47	46	45	44	43	42	41	31	32	33	34	35	36	37	38

Mandibular right   Mandibular left

Deciduous Dentition

Maxillary right   Maxillary left

55	54	53	52	51	61	62	63	64	65
85	84	83	82	81	71	72	73	74	75

Mandibular right   Mandibular left

Zsigmond System

Permanent Dentition

Maxillary right   Maxillary left

8	7	6	5	4	3	2	1	1	2	3	4	5	6	7	8
8	7	6	5	4	3	2	1	1	2	3	4	5	6	7	8

Mandibular right   Mandibular left

Deciduous Dentition

Maxillary right   Maxillary left

$$E \quad D \quad C \quad B \quad A \mid A \quad B \quad C \quad D \quad E$$

$$E \quad D \quad C \quad B \quad A \mid A \quad B \quad C \quad D \quad E$$

Mandibular right   Mandibular left

In all cases, and regardless of which system of shorthand is used, the only sure method to minimize mistakes is a full description including the five considerations for each tooth, as previously discussed. This is of obvious clinical importance, especially when teeth are to be extracted, and many clinicians use special abbreviations is order to describe a tooth fully, which are derived from Latin. For those unfortunate enough not to have been blessed with the inestimable benefits of a classical education,[1] these are listed below together with their full Latin and English names:

| | | Abbreviation | |
| | | Deciduous | Permanent |
English name	*Latin name*	*Dentition*	*Dentition*
First or central incisor	Incisivus primus	i_1	I_1
Second incisor	Incisivus secundus	i_2	I_2
Canine or cuspid	Caninus or cuspidatus	c	C
First premolar or bicuspid	Praemolaris primus	—	P_1
Second premolar or bicuspid	Praemolaris secundus	—	P_2
First molar	Molaris primus	m_1	M_1
Second molar	Molaris secundus	m_2	M_2
Third molar	Molaris tertius	—	M_3
Upper right	Superior dexter	sd	
Upper left	Superior sinister	ss	
Lower right	Inferior dexter	id	
Lower left	Inferior sinister	is	

[1] With apologies to D.J.A.

Collecting and Preserving Extracted Teeth

In order to be able to study tooth morphology thoroughly, it is advisable for the student to have his own personal collection of extracted teeth at his disposal.

It takes most general dental practitioners at least 6 months to fill a small jar with reasonably sound extracted teeth (and then usually first premolars and third molars) and for this reason the student should not wait until the last minute in writing to his dentist, and neighbouring practitioners in his home town, for help. In general, practices in the vicinity of a dental school should not be approached since they most probably already have an agreement to supply directly to the university.

A short telephone call to the dentist concerned is unlikely to be fruitful, especially during busy surgery hours. Much better results are achieved if the student makes an appointment to introduce himself personally to the dentist, or failing this, a written request. A personal visit is preferable since this enables the student to supply the dentist with a suitable container for the teeth. Ideally, this should be made of a strong, opaque plastic with an easily removable lid, and a neat label on the outside with the student's name, address and telephone number printed clearly thereon. It should be half filled with a 10 per cent solution of household bleach in water. If the dentist himself has to hunt around the practice for a suitable empty jar, the request is most likely to be forgotten.

Other preservatives may also be used, such as formalin, or 1 per cent phenol in water, although in the author's experience, and without wishing to make this sound like an advertisement for toothpaste, diluted bleach gives the best results— the teeth remain relatively odour-free and also become cleaner and whiter.

In order to remove remnants of bone, calculus or gingiva, the teeth should be rinsed and placed in a stronger solution of approximately 30 per cent household bleach for a few days.

Stubborn remnants of bone or calculus can be removed with an old knife or wood chisel, scraping *carefully away* from the fingers whilst resting the tooth on a piece of scrap wood. (This is not to be compared with scraping potatoes, and furthermore, a full complement of fingers is desirable for the student's future career!)

After the teeth have all been satisfactorily cleaned, they may be kept in a fresh solution of 10 per cent household bleach in water. It is important that the teeth are kept wet for use at a later stage in a phantom head. Dry teeth fracture very easily and are therefore unsuitable for cavity preparations. Moreover, the chance of a neat cleavage of the tooth with a chisel is greater if the tooth has been kept wet. This is of relevance in the study of endodontic anatomy (*see* 'Introduction', Endodontic Anatomy, page 99).

Section 1

The Deciduous Dentition

The deciduous, primary, or, as they are often referred to colloquially, 'milk' teeth, have a relatively short life-span before they are exfoliated (shed) to be replaced by the permanent teeth. This usually occurs between the ages of 6 and 13 years. The deciduous incisors and canines have permanent successors but the first and second deciduous molars are replaced by the first and second premolars respectively.

The deciduous dentition comprises fewer teeth than the permanent dentition with a total of 10 maxillary and 10 mandibular teeth. They are as follows, in order of position from the mandible (the corresponding dental shorthand is also given):

A   First incisor
B   Second incisor
C   Canine
D   First molar
E   Second molar

The shorthand dental formula for the deciduous dentition is as follows:

$$DI\frac{2}{2}DC\frac{1}{1}DM\frac{2}{2} = 10$$

The deciduous teeth have several important differences in morphology, composition, size, colour etc., and these are listed below.

Principal Differences Between Deciduous and Permanent Teeth

1. The deciduous teeth are smaller overall than the permanent teeth.
2. The enamel of the deciduous teeth is whiter and more opaque, which gives the crown a lighter colour than that of the permanent teeth.
3. The enamel of the deciduous teeth is more permeable and more easily worn down. The degree of permeability is lessened after the start of root resorption.
4. The depth of enamel is more consistent and thinner than in the permanent teeth, being from 0·5 mm to 1·00 mm thick. The enamel of permanent teeth is approximately 2·5 mm thick.
5. Deciduous teeth have a pronounced cervical margin. The enamel bulges, instead of tapering gently, at the cemento-enamel junction, in much the same way that the stomach of an obese gentleman protrudes beyond his swimming trunks. This cervical bulge is accentuated in the mesiobuccal area of deciduous molars.
6. The crowns of anterior deciduous teeth are bulbous, with a pronounced labial cingulum.
7. In newly-erupted deciduous teeth the cusps tend to be more pointed.
8. The roots of deciduous teeth are shorter, less strong and lighter in colour than those of the permanent teeth.
9. The roots of anterior deciduous teeth are longer in proportion to the crown. The roots of posterior teeth are more divergent to allow for the developing permanent successor. They flare out from each other wider than the crown measurement, and from a minimal common root trunk.

10. The pulp chambers are larger than in the permanent teeth with prominent pulp horns, and follow the exterior morphology of the tooth more closely. There tends, correspondingly to be less depth of dentine.
11. The root canals of deciduous teeth are very fine.
12. The deciduous teeth display a more constant morphology than the permanent teeth, with fewer variations.
13. The cemento-enamel junction of deciduous teeth is less sinuous than in permanent teeth.
14. The deciduous dentition comprises 20 teeth; the permanent dentition comprises 32.

Endodontic anatomy of the deciduous teeth, *see* page 103.

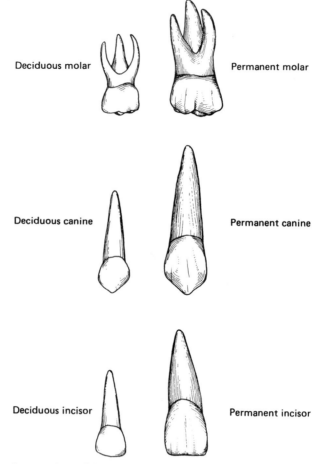

Deciduous molar — Permanent molar

Deciduous canine — Permanent canine

Deciduous incisor — Permanent incisor

Fig. 6. A comparison of the exterior morphology of deciduous teeth with that of the permanent teeth.

Deciduous Maxillary Dental Arch

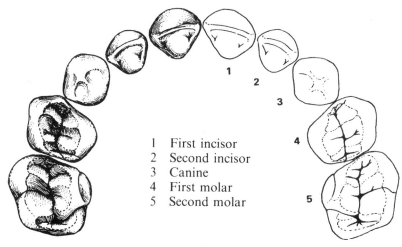

1   First incisor
2   Second incisor
3   Canine
4   First molar
5   Second molar

Fig. 7.

Deciduous Mandibular Dental Arch

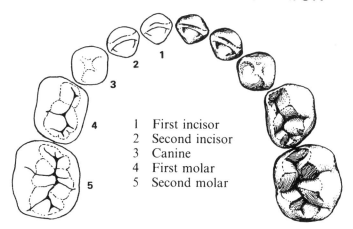

1   First incisor
2   Second incisor
3   Canine
4   First molar
5   Second molar

Fig. 8.

13

Maxillary First Deciduous Incisor

Chronology

Initial calcification: 3–4 months in utero.
Completion of crown: 4 months.
Eruption: $7\frac{1}{2}$ months.
Completion of root: $1\frac{1}{2}$ years.

General

The maxillary central deciduous incisors occupy the central space on either side of the midline of the maxilla. The crown and root form is essentially the same as that of the maxillary first permanent incisor but on a slightly smaller scale, and, for this reason, it is very helpful to compare the two teeth in order to notice their differences.

The most obvious feature of the deciduous incisor is the increased mesiodistal width of the crown, which exceeds its cervico-incisal length; the opposite is true of the permanent successor, in which the crown is proportionately longer. This does not affect its typical incisor morphology, however. The crown is basically shovel-shaped with ill-defined marginal ridges and a straight incisive edge which is centred over the bulk of the crown.

Although the crown of the first permanent incisor is described as 'stout in appearance', it does not have the round, fuller shape of the maxillary first deciduous incisor. From the mesial and distal aspects, the crown appears relatively broad, labiopalatally, because of the bulbous labial surface and the greater convexity of the large palatal cingulum which extends almost to the incisive edge and which occupies most of the otherwise concave palatal surface. These more rounded contours, which are characteristic of all the deciduous teeth, are accentuated near the cervix where the crown appears to bulge out at the base as it sits on the root. The cervical margin itself shows its greatest sinuosity on the mesial side and to a lesser extent on the distal.

From the labial aspect the crown shows an exaggerated characteristic of the upper first permanent incisor: the differences between the mesial and distal corners of the incisive edge are very definite in that the disto-incisal angle is well-rounded compared with the sharper mesio-incisal angle. No grooves or depressions are present on the labial surface.

The root is longer in proportion to the crown than in the permanent central incisor, and tapers elegantly to a rather blunt apex and exhibits a slight distal inclination. In cross-section it is roughly circular and slightly flattened on the labial and palatal surfaces. Mamelons are rarely seen in the incisive edge of the newly erupted deciduous incisors.

Principal Identifying Features

1. *Rounded disto-incisal angle: sharp mesio-incisal angle.*
2. *Crown similar to upper first permanent incisor but smaller and plumper overall.*

3. Large palatal cingulum and pronounced bulge on labial surface.
4. Root tilts distally and slightly labially from long axis of crown, and tapers to a blunt apex.
5. The mesiodistal and cervico-incisal dimensions of the crown are nearly the same in the unworn specimen.

Variations

No noticeable variations.

I_1 superior, *see* page 49.
Endodontic anatomy, *see* page 105.

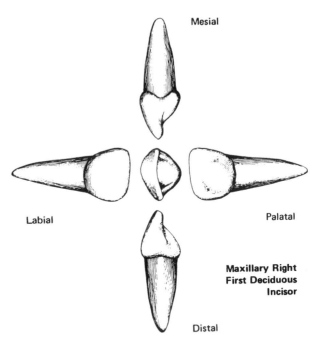

Mesial

Labial

Palatal

Distal

**Maxillary Right
First Deciduous
Incisor**

Fig. 9.

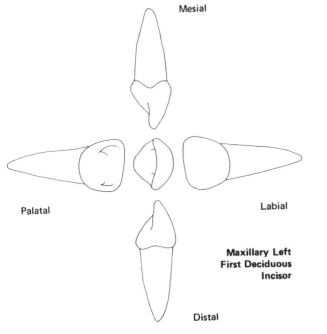

Mesial

Palatal

Labial

Distal

**Maxillary Left
First Deciduous
Incisor**

Fig. 10.

17

Mandibular First Deciduous Incisor

Chronology

Initial calcification: $4\frac{1}{2}$ months in utero.
Completion of crown: 4 months.
Eruption: $6\frac{1}{2}$ months.
Completion of root: $1\frac{1}{2}$–2 years.

General

The mandibular first deciduous incisor occupies the central space on either side of the midline of the mandible. It has a typical, chisel-shaped incisor morphology with a wedge-shaped crown rising to a thin, straight incisive edge centred over the long axis of the tooth, when viewed from the mesial or distal aspects.

From the incisal aspect the crown has a rounded triangular outline formed by a wide labial surface, and the mesial and distal surfaces which converge onto the narrower curvature of the lingual surface.

The lingual surface, although essentially concave, is partially filled with a well-developed lingual cingulum. It is bounded on the proximal surfaces by marginal ridges which are less prominent than those of the maxillary deciduous incisors, or those of the permanent successors.

There is a marked bulge of the crown at the cervix, as in all deciduous teeth, and the crown, as a whole, is smaller and chubbier than that of the mandibular first permanent incisor. It is less angular, with a symmetrical outline, and appears wider in proportion to its length, although the root is approximately twice as long as the crown. This gives the tooth a slender appearance.

The mandibular first deciduous incisor is easily distinguished from its larger distal neighbour; their difference in size is more obvious than that of their permanent successors: the mandibular second deciduous incisor is much larger. The symmetry of the crown makes it almost impossible to distinguish left from right in isolated specimens, but a helpful clue is that the cervical margin rises further towards the incisive edge on the mesial than on the distal surface, and if a root is present, it will tend to incline distally.

Compared with the mesiodistally flattened roots of the mandibular permanent incisors, the root is more rounded in cross-section.

Principal Identifying Features

1. *Single tapered root more rounded than that of mandibular first permanent incisor. Tends to incline distally.*
2. *Smallest tooth in the deciduous dentition.*
3. Cervical margin most sinuous on mesial side.
4. Bulge on labial surface at cemento-enamel junction.
5. Chisel-shaped crown.

18

Variations

The pronounced cervical bulge on the labial surface may be reduced or completely absent.

I_1 inferior, *see* page 52.
Endodontic anatomy, *see* page 105.

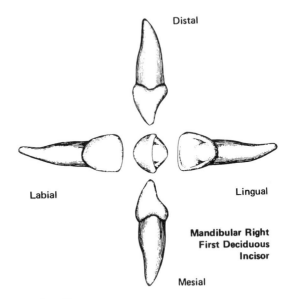

Distal

Labial

Lingual

**Mandibular Right
First Deciduous
Incisor**

Mesial

Fig. 11.

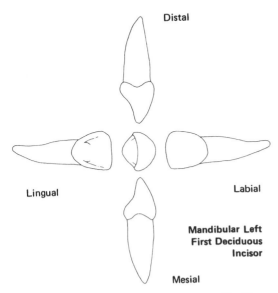

Distal

Lingual

Labial

**Mandibular Left
First Deciduous
Incisor**

Mesial

Fig. 12.

19

Maxillary Second Deciduous Incisor

Chronology

Initial calcification: $4\frac{1}{2}$ months in utero.
Completion of crown: 5 months.
Eruption: 8–9 months.
Completion of root: $1\frac{1}{2}$–2 years.

General

The maxillary lateral deciduous incisor is situated second from the midline of the maxilla and is similar in its morphology to the upper central incisor, which it supplements in the function of cutting food. The crown is not as long, proportionately, as that of its permanent successor, but resembles that of the first deciduous incisor in having a greater mesiodistal width. In most cases, this width does not exceed the cervico-incisal length but is approximately equal to it. Worn specimens will, of course, show a proportionately wider crown.

The crown is smaller than that of the maxillary deciduous central incisor in all dimensions, but otherwise the two may be difficult to tell apart, if studied individually, instead of comparatively, as they have a greater similarity than the same teeth of the permanent dentition. One important difference, however, is that the lingual cingulum is not as prominent in the lateral incisor. This same situation exists in the maxillary permanent incisors although the maxillary lateral deciduous incisor never encloses a pit or foramen caecum incisivum on the palatal surface.

The incisive edge is straight and placed centrally over the crown. It slopes from the mesial to the, slightly shorter, distal surface where it merges into the rounded disto-incisal angle, in contrast with the sharp mesio-incisal angle.

The root is similar in all respects to that of the maxillary first deciduous incisor with the same narrow cervix and blunt apex, but is slightly longer in proportion to the crown. The problem with all the deciduous teeth is in finding a specimen with its root intact because, in the majority of cases, the tooth is shed only when the root has been almost completely resorbed by the permanent successor. An indication of the root lengths is therefore often best seen radiographically. This stresses the importance of a good knowledge of the crown morphology when identifying deciduous teeth.

Principal Identifying Features

1. *Similar shape to maxillary first deciduous incisor but crown smaller and narrower in proportion.*
2. *Palatal cingulum less pronounced.*
3. Rounded disto-incisal angle; sharp mesio-incisal angle.
4. Single root.

Variations

Rare, in contrast with the highly variable maxillary second permanent incisor.
I_2 superior, *see* page 55.
Endodontic anatomy, *see* page 105.

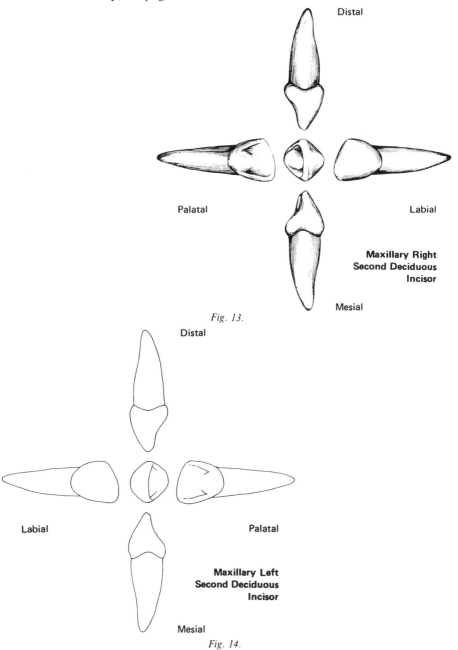

Distal

Palatal

Labial

Maxillary Right Second Deciduous Incisor

Mesial

Fig. 13.

Distal

Labial

Palatal

Maxillary Left Second Deciduous Incisor

Mesial

Fig. 14.

Mandibular Second Deciduous Incisor

Chronology

Initial calcification $4\frac{1}{2}$ months in utero.
Completion of crown: $4\frac{1}{2}$ months.
Eruption: 7 months.
Completion of root: $1\frac{1}{2}$–2 years.

General

The mandibular second deciduous incisor is situated second from the midline of the mandible and supplements the function of the central incisor in cutting food. It is very similar to the mandibular second permanent incisor, in its general form, but differs in the usual characteristics of deciduous teeth, such as the pronounced bulge of the crown at the cervix and a plumper shape overall with smaller, rounded contours.

It is easy to tell to which side of the mandible it belongs, because, from the labial aspect, the disto-incisal angle is rounded, compared with a much sharper, often acute, mesio-incisal angle. Unfortunately this feature, with the incisive edge sloping down towards the slightly shorter distal surface, is also found in the maxillary second deciduous incisor, which often causes the two to be confused, especially since they are about the same size. The only difference between them is the larger cingulum on the lingual surface of the mandibular second deciduous incisor. This does not increase its labiolingual thickness, however, which is approximately the same as that of the smaller mandibular first deciduous incisor.

In some cases, the apparent twisting of the crown on the root to enable the incisive edge to follow the curve of the mandibular arch, as found in the mandibular second permanent incisor, is faintly discernible.

The single root is not flattened mesiodistally, like that of its permanent successor, but more rounded, so that in cross-section it is almost circular. It tends to curve distally.

Principal Identifying Features

1. *Rounded disto-incisal angle; sharp mesio-incisal angle.*
2. *Single tapered root with round cross-section, tends to incline distally.*
3. Incisive edge slopes downwards from medial to slightly lower distal surface in unworn examples.
4. Crown may, in some cases, show twisting on root in order to allow the incisive edge to follow the mandibular arch.
5. Larger than mandibular first deciduous incisor.
6. Lingual surface may be more concave than that of the mandibular first deciduous incisor.
7. Single root which is generally longer than that of the mandibular first deciduous incisor.

Variations

No noticeable variations. A feature of the deciduous dentition is its consistency in its morphology.

I_2 inferior, *see* page 58.
Endodontic anatomy, *see* page 105.

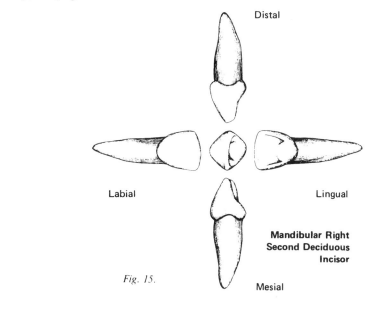

Distal

Labial   Lingual

**Mandibular Right
Second Deciduous
Incisor**

Fig. 15.

Mesial

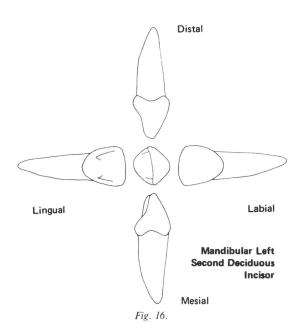

Distal

Lingual   Labial

**Mandibular Left
Second Deciduous
Incisor**

Mesial

Fig. 16.

23

Maxillary Deciduous Canine

Chronology

Initial calcification: 5 months in utero.
Completion of crown: 9 months.
Eruption: 16–20 months.
Completion of root: approximately 3 years.

General

The maxillary deciduous canine is the third tooth from the midline of the maxilla. Although the overall size of the tooth is smaller, it is sometimes easily confused with the permanent canine because of its large crown and stout labiolingual proportions.

Because the root is *proportionately* longer than that of the maxillary permanent canine, the upper deciduous canine has a more slender appearance except for the plump crown which has an accentuated bulge at the constricted cervical margin, and a relatively large mesiodistal width typical of anterior teeth in the deciduous dentition. The crown is more or less symmetrically cone-shaped and surmounted by a sharp cusp tip which soon wears down with use. The contact areas on the proximal surfaces are at approximately the same level. In contrast to the maxillary permanent canine, if asymmetry is present in the crown of the upper deciduous canine than it is the *mesial* rather than the *distal* slope which is the longer.

The palatal surface is strongly convex with a well-developed cingulum and mesial and distal marginal ridges. Confluent with the cingulum is a ridge which extends to the cusp tip. The same ridge formation is present on the convex labial surface and connects the labial bulge at the cervical third of the crown with the cusp tip. Sometimes, a shallow groove may be seen running longitudinally along either side of it.

From the incisal aspect the crown outline is approximately diamond-shaped with rounded corners, compared with the more circular outline shown by the maxillary permanent canine from this aspect. The corners of the diamond are formed by the mesial and distal contact points, and by the prominent lingual and labial ridges which run from the cusp tip to the centres of the lingual and labial bulges respectively, so that although the crown is basically conical, it also has four flattened surfaces.

The root is approximately twice or more the length of the crown, and has a well-rounded triangular cross-section similar to that of the maxillary permanent canine, with labial, distopalatal and mesiopalatal surfaces. It has a slender taper and tends to incline distally.

Principal Identifying Features

1. *Mesial slope of longer than distal slope.*
2. *Conical crown with pronounced cervical bulge and pointed cusp.*
3. *Crown smaller and more bulbous than that of the upper permanent canine.*

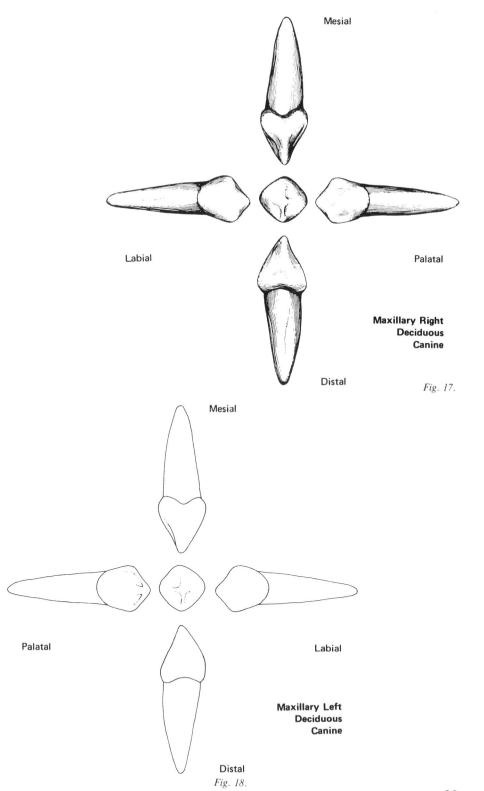

Mesial

Labial

Palatal

**Maxillary Right
Deciduous
Canine**

Distal

Fig. 17.

Mesial

Palatal

Labial

**Maxillary Left
Deciduous
Canine**

Distal

Fig. 18.

25

4. Labial and palatal longitudinal ridges extending from cusp tip.
5. The incisal aspect displays a diamond-shaped outline with rounded corners from incisal aspect.
6. Cervical margin extends further incisally on the mesial surface than on the distal surface.
7. Slender tapering single root often more than twice the length of the crown with a tendency to incline distally. Cross-section similar to that of the maxillary permanent canine.

Variations

Asymmetrical and symmetrical crown forms are equally common. An occasional variation is the flattening or partial bifurcation of the labial surface of the root, resulting in a longitudinal labial groove and a heart-shaped cross-section of the root.

C superior, *see* page 61.
Endodontic anatomy, *see* page 106.

Mandibular Deciduous Canine

Chronology

Initial calcification: 5 months in utero.
Completion of crown: 9 months.
Eruption: 16–20 months.
Completion of root: $2\frac{1}{2}$–3 years.

General

The mandibular deciduous canine is the third tooth from the midline of the mandible. It is much plumper than the mandibular permanent canine with exaggerated mesial and distal convexities, which give the crown rather wider mediodistal proportions. These same differences occur between the maxillary deciduous and permanent canines, and are characteristics typical of anterior deciduous teeth.

From the occlusal aspect, the mandibular deciduous canine shows the rounded diamond-shaped coronal outline found in the maxillary deciduous canine, but to a lesser degree, which gives it an outline form which also resembles that of the mandibular deciduous incisors. This is because the labiolingual thickness of the crown is greatly reduced in proportion to that of the maxillary deciduous canine, with much less pronounced labial and lingual cervical ridges, giving it a more slender appearance. The lingual longitudinal ridge is scarcely discernible, and, as a consequence, the lingual surface is concave with its only convexity being that of its cingulum.

When once it is established that the specimen being studied is a mandibular, and not a maxillary deciduous canine, by virtue of the factors discussed above, its provenance is easily determined: from the labial aspect the distal slope appears longer than the mesial. This is a similar arrangement to that of the permanent canines, but it is reversed in the maxillary deciduous canine when asymmetry is present.

The mesial and distal aspects give a less obvious clue; the cervical margin rises slightly farther incisally on the mesial side than on the distal.

The mandibular deciduous canine has a single root with a rounded triangular cross-section similar to that of the maxillary deciduous canine. It inclines distally and slightly labially.

Principal Identifying Features

1. *Smaller and slimmer overall than the maxillary deciduous canine.*
2. *Distal slope longer than mesial.*
3. Concave lingual surface.
4. Less well-defined labial and lingual longitudinal ridges; lingual ridge often completely absent.
5. Cervical margin more sinuous on mesial side.
6. Single tapering root inclines distally and slightly labially.

Variations

No noticeable variations. Lingual longitudinal ridge occasionally present on lingual surface.

C inferior, *see* page 64.
Endodontic anatomy, *see* page 106.

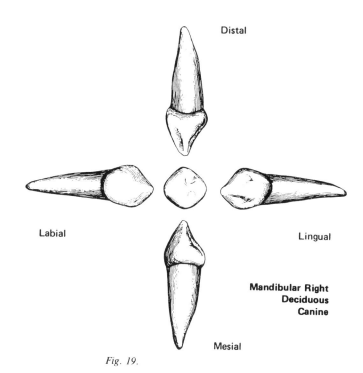

Distal

Labial

Lingual

**Mandibular Right
Deciduous
Canine**

Mesial

Fig. 19.

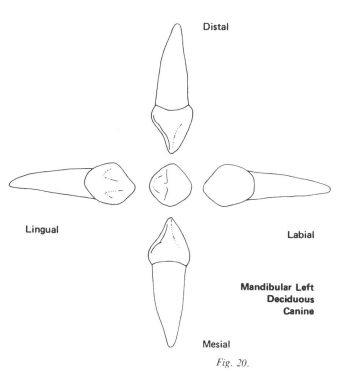

Distal

Lingual

Labial

**Mandibular Left
Deciduous
Canine**

Mesial

Fig. 20.

29

Maxillary First Deciduous Molar

Chronology

Initial calcification: 5 months in utero.
Completion of crown: 6 months.
Eruption: 12–16 months.
Completion of roots: 2–2½ years.

General

When viewed from the occlusal aspect, the crown of this tooth is seen to be clearly divided into a buccal and lingual half by a deep central developmental fissure which runs mesiodistally connecting the mesial, central and distal fossae. Each half consists of a large cusp with a smaller accessory cusp distal to it, but which, nevertheless, is regarded as a cusp in its own right. The upper first deciduous molar therefore has four cusps: mesiopalatal, mesiobuccal, distobuccal and distopalatal, in decreasing order of size and development.

The combined mesiodistal width of the two lingual cusps is less than that of the two buccal cusps, which results in a trapezoid coronal outline with its widest dimension mesiodistally, and an obtuse mesiopalatal angle when viewed from the occlusal aspect. This is accentuated in the three-cusped form which sometimes occurs, when the lingual developmental groove, and hence the distopalatal cusp, is absent. The cusps appear more as ridges running mesiodistally, which, when combined with the mesial and distal marginal ridges, enclose the occlusal surface within a roughly rectangular, cup-shaped area that is compressed in the buccopalatal direction. The crown converges palatally from its wide cervical bulge to the narrow occlusal surface, and is widest labiopalatally towards the mesial surface.

The views from the mesial and distal aspects both show the crown to have a pronounced bulge near the cervix, particularly on the mesial side of the buccal surface. This convexity, which sits on and extends a millimetre or so down the mesiobuccal root, is sometimes developed to the extent that it is hemispherical. It is the main feature of the first deciduous molars and is sometimes referred to as the 'molar tubercle of Zuckerkandl'.

The mesial and distal surfaces of the crown do not have a cervical bulge, but flare out from the cervix to the mesial and distal marginal ridges.

The upper first deciduous molar has three roots with similar morphology and positions to those of the other maxillary molars, i.e. two buccal and one palatal, but they arise directly from the cervix and not from a common root trunk. They are the palatal, mesiobuccal and distobuccal, in descending order of size and divergence, although they all diverge markedly, except for the apices which tend to converge again, giving the roots the appearance of a crane-grab. The buccal roots are sometimes partially fused together.

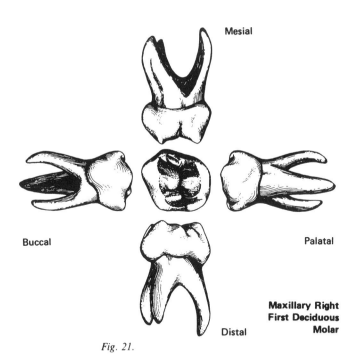

Mesial

Buccal

Palatal

Distal

**Maxillary Right
First Deciduous
Molar**

Fig. 21.

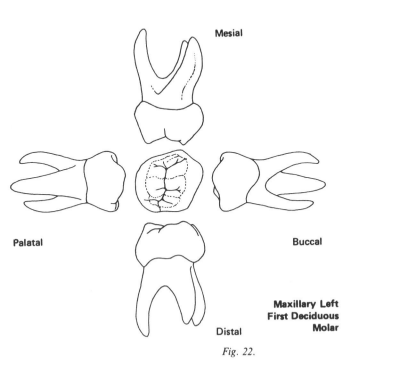

Mesial

Palatal

Buccal

Distal

**Maxillary Left
First Deciduous
Molar**

Fig. 22.

31

Principal Identifying Features

1. *Pronounced bulge on mesial side of buccal surface: molar tubercle of Zuckerkandl.*
2. *Trapezoid coronal outline with narrow occlusal surface running mesiodistally.*
3. Palatal surface shorter, mediodistally, than the buccal surface.
4. Mesiopalatal cusp largest and most pointed.
5. Widest labiopalatal crown measurement at mesial end.
6. Three widely divergent roots.

Variations

Palatal and distobuccal roots sometimes fuse.
Mesiobuccal cusp sometimes has an accessory cusp mesial to it.
Distopalatal cusp sometimes absent.
Zuckerkandl's tubercle is occasionally scarcely discernible.

M_1 superior, *see* page 79.
Endodontic anatomy, *see* page 106.

Mandibular First Deciduous Molar

Chronology

Initial calcification: 5 months in utero.
Completion of crown: 6 months.
Eruption: 12–16 months.
Completion of roots: 2–$2\frac{1}{2}$ years.

General

From the occlusal aspect, the coronal outline of the mandibular first deciduous molar is irregularly quadrilateral with a longer mediodistal measurement than buccolingual.

The lingually inclined occlusal surface comprises four cusps: two prominent buccal cusps and two smaller lingual cusps. The buccal cusps are compressed labiolingually to the extent that they are placed approximately centrally along the mesiodistal diameter of the coronal outline. The mesiobuccal cusp is more prominent that the distobuccal, and they are separated only by a shallow depression, rather than a developmental groove as found in the other mandibular molars, so that the buccal surface is completely smooth. Joining the two mesial cusps is a ridge of enamel called the 'buccolingual crest', which has a small fossa mesial to it and a longer one distal to it. Occasionally, when this ridge is poorly developed or even absent, there is a continuous central developmental fissure resulting in a shallow cup-shaped occlusal surface. The fissure runs mesiodistally separating the buccal and lingual cusps along the length of the occlusal surface, and ends at the marginal ridges, winding around the bases of the cusps in a zig-zag pattern.

The two lingual cusps are roughly conical in shape, and their combined mesiodistal width is less than that of the buccal cusps. The mesiolingual cusp is always larger than the distolingual which is occasionally reduced to the extent that it appears only to be an accessory cusplet on the distal arm of the mesiolingual cusp.

The main distinguishing feature of the mandibular first deciduous molar is the extremely well-developed bulge of the large, lingually-inclined buccal surface, and because of this the cervical constriction appears to be quite considerable in this tooth. This distension is often developed to a distinct hemispherical protuberance near the cervical margin on the mesial part of the buccal surface, over the mesial root, and is referred to as the 'molar tubercle of Zuckerkandl'. A similar tubercle is present on the maxillary first deciduous molar.

There are two roots positioned similarly to those of the other mandibular molars, i.e. one mesial and one distal. They are flattened mesiodistally, particularly the mesial root, in much the same way as those of the mandibular first permanent molar, but diverge more, however, in order to make room for the underlying first premolar. The mesial root tapers very little and appears rectangular in shape, with an apical ridge rather than a tapered point. It is longer than the distal root.

Principal Identifying Features

1. *Molar tubercle of Zuckerkandl an exaggerated cervical bulge on the buccal surface of the crown over the mesial root, with a considerable cervical constriction.*
2. *Four cusps: buccal cusps compressed labiolingually with no clear separation between them in contrast to the two lingual cusps which are clearly defined and roughly conical in shape.*
3. Mesiobuccal cusp largest.
4. Tooth longer mediodistally than labiolingually.
5. Mesial marginal ridge more pronounced than distal.
6. Two roots flattened mesiodistally. The mesial is the longer and from the mesial aspect appears rectangular, and is often grooved.

Variations

Distolingual cusp sometimes very insignificant.
Buccolingual crest occasionally absent.

M_1 inferior, *see* page 82.
Endodontic anatomy *see* page 106.

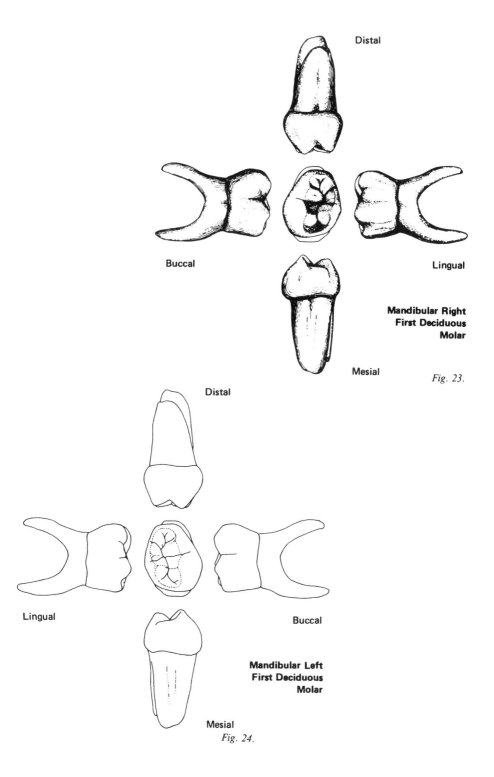

Distal

Buccal

Lingual

**Mandibular Right
First Deciduous
Molar**

Mesial

Fig. 23.

Distal

Lingual

Buccal

**Mandibular Left
First Deciduous
Molar**

Mesial

Fig. 24.

35

Maxillary Second Deciduous Molar

Chronology

Initial calcification: 6 months in utero.
Completion of crown: 10–12 months.
Eruption: $1\frac{3}{4}$–$2\frac{1}{2}$ years.
Completion of roots: 3 years.

General

The maxillary second deciduous molar is the fifth and last tooth from the midline of the maxilla, in the deciduous dentition.

Not much more can be said about this tooth than has been mentioned already in the description of the maxillary first permanent molar, of which it is almost an exact replica but to a smaller scale. Its deciduous characteristics, however, make it necessary to describe the main identifying features of this tooth in order to distinguish it from the other deciduous molars.

It is very helpful to compare the maxillary second deciduous molar with a specimen of a maxillary first permanent molar in order to appreciate more fully their subtle differences, as follows: the three roots are similarly placed but are more slender and have a wider divergence than those of the maxillary first permanent molar in order to make room for the developing maxillary second premolar; the crown of the maxillary second deciduous molar has a more prominent bulge on the cervical part of the buccal surface than the upper first permanent molar, but this is never developed to the extent of the molar tubercle of Zuckerkandl present in the upper first deciduous molar.

The maxillary second deciduous molar has four cusps, the mesiopalatal being the most prominent. This is joined to the distobuccal cusp by an oblique ridge, an important characteristic present in the maxillary permanent molars.

Since the maxillary second deciduous molar is almost an exact copy of the maxillary first permanent molar, the unique feature of the cusp of Carabelli, which is frequently present on the palatal surface of the mesiopalatal cusp, is also duplicated. In fact, it occurs in a greater proportion of cases in the maxillary second deciduous molar.

Principal Identifying Features

1. *Morphology of maxillary first permanent molar duplicated on a smaller scale.*
2. *More prominent bulge on cervical part of buccal surface.*
3. Three roots.
4. Roots have wider divergence than those of maxillary first permanent molar.
5. Cusp of Carabelli present in most cases.

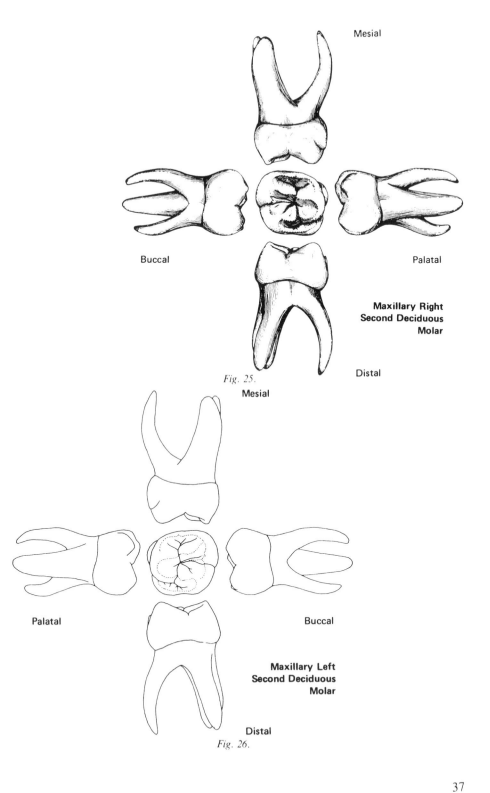

Mesial

Buccal

Palatal

**Maxillary Right
Second Deciduous
Molar**

Fig. 25.

Distal

Mesial

Palatal

Buccal

**Maxillary Left
Second Deciduous
Molar**

Distal

Fig. 26.

Variations

Cusp of Carabelli may be absent
Very rarely the distopalatal cusp may be so reduced as to be scarcely discernible.
The two buccal roots may sometimes by partially fused.

M_1 superior, *see* page 79.
M_2 superior, *see* page 85.
Endodontic anatomy, *see* page 106.

Mandibular Second Deciduous Molar

Chronology

Initial calcification: 6 months in utero.
Completion of crown: 10–12 months.
Eruption: $1\frac{3}{4}$–$2\frac{1}{2}$ years.
Completion of roots: 3 years.

General

This is the fifth and last tooth from the midline of the mandible, and is similar to the mandibular first permanent molar in its general morphology although it is smaller in proportion. The resemblance is not as close as that of the maxillary second deciduous molar and the maxillary first permanent molar because the deciduous characteristics of the mandibular second deciduous molar are more pronounced.

From the occlusal aspect five cusps can be seen, three buccal and two lingual, and these are in the same arrangement as those of the mandibular first permanent molar. The coronal outline is similar in that the mesiodistal width is greater than the buccolingual. The three buccal cusps, however, are practically all the same reduced size so that the mesiodistal width of the buccal surface, although still slightly greater than that of the lingual surface, is accordingly reduced in proportion to that of the mandibular first permanent molar. From the occlusal aspect this gives the crown a comparatively more regular rectangular outline. Due to the more equal size of the buccal cusps, the pattern of the central developmental fissure is altered slightly so that the bases of the mesiolingual and centrobuccal cusps rarely meet at the central fossa. This would otherwise give the primitive *Dryopithecus* pattern that is so commonly present in the mandibular first permanent molars.

Another feature found in the mandibular first permanent molar but not in the mandibular second deciduous molar is the difference in the number of cusps visible when the crown is viewed from the buccal and lingual aspects. Because the lingual cusps are more conical in shape and the separation between them is slightly deeper than in the mandibular first permanent molar, all five cusps are usually visible from both the buccal and lingual aspects. From these aspects other important comparative characteristics of the mandibular second deciduous molar are visible: the mesial and distal surfaces flare out to a more notable extent from a relatively narrow cervix to the strongly convex proximal contact areas, whereas the cervical part of the lingually inclined buccal surface has a greater bulge than that of the mandibular first permanent molar.

As in the mandibular first permanent molar, the mandibular second deciduous molar has two roots which are long, slender and flattened mesiodistally. There is hardly any common root trunk, especially on the buccal side where the bifurcation of the roots occurs just below the cervical margin. The roots are widely divergent, a characteristic of all the deciduous molars, and the apices may sometimes converge again. The mesial root is longer and more flattened than the distal. From the mesial aspect it is roughly rectangular in outline with a flat, blunt apex and a tendency sometimes to subdivide into a buccal and lingual root.

Principal Identifying Features

1. *Same arrangement of cusps and roots as the mandibular first permanent molar.*
2. *Smaller and whiter than lower first permanent molar but larger than the mandibular first deciduous molar.*
3. *Prominent cervical bulge on buccal surface of crown.* Buccal surface inclined lingually.
4. Occlusal outline rectangular.
5. Buccal cusps approximately equal in size.
6. Two widely divergent roots; mesial root longer and flattened mesiodistally.

Variation

Partial diversion of mesial root may sometimes be present.

M$_1$ inferior, *see* page 82.
M$_2$ inferior, *see* page 88.
Endodontic anatomy, *see* page 106.

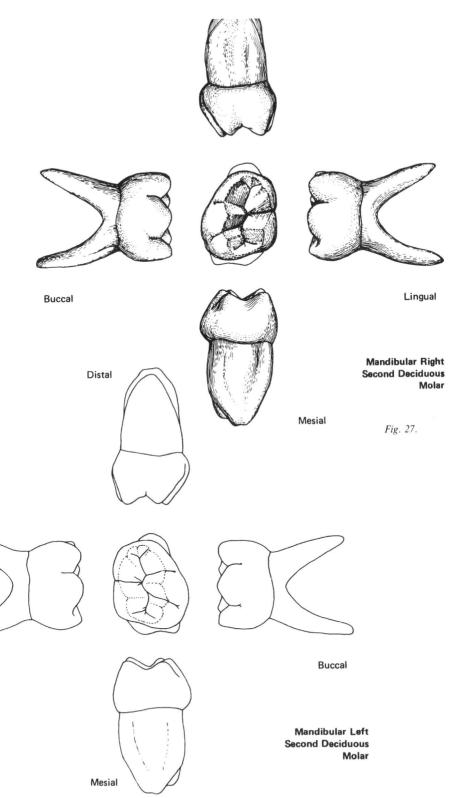

Buccal

Lingual

Distal

Mesial

**Mandibular Right
Second Deciduous
Molar**

Fig. 27.

Lingual

Buccal

Mesial

**Mandibular Left
Second Deciduous
Molar**

Fig. 28.

41

Section 2

The Permanent Dentition

The full complement of teeth in the permanent dentition is 32, 16 teeth in either jaw. Starting from the midline and progressing posteriorly, they are as follows (the corresponding dental shorthand is also given):

1 Central incisor
2 Lateral incisor
3 Canine
4 First premolar
5 Second premolar
6 First molar
7 Second molar
8 Third molar

The shorthand dental formula for the permanent dentition is as follows:

$$I\frac{2}{2}C\frac{1}{1}P\frac{2}{2}M\frac{3}{3} = 16$$

The Permanent Incisors

There are four incisors in the maxilla and four in the mandible, and they are situated centrally with two incisors on either side of the midline, so that they function together in cutting and shearing food into small pieces suitable for mastication. They are also aesthetically very important teeth.

The maxillary incisors are larger than the mandibular incisors with a conical, tapering root and a crown that is relatively wider mesiodistally. The roots of the mandibular incisors are flattened mesiodistally with a blunter apex.

The incisors of both the upper and lower jaws are named according to their position from the midline. Those centred on either side of the midline are called the 'first' or 'central' incisors, and the second from the midline are known either as 'lateral' or as 'second' incisors. Also common to the maxillary and mandibular incisors is the typical incisor form which is essentially chisel-shaped with a wedge-shaped crown outline when viewed from the mesial or distal aspects. Unworn, newly-erupted specimens of incisor teeth have three small mamelons or bumps on the incisive edge which are soon worn to a flat edge after masticatory use.

The cervical margin of all the incisors is very sinuous and rises towards the incisive edge on the mesial and distal surfaces. The mesial rise is much higher than that on the distal surface.

Well-developed marginal ridges sometimes give the maxillary incisors a 'shovel-shaped' appearance and this variation of the palatal surface occurs most commonly in certain communities, namely among the Mongoloid and American Indian peoples.

The Permanent Canines

The function of the canines is to grip and tear food. It is the last of the anterior group of teeth and is situated third from the midline in the 'corners' of the dental arch between the anterior and buccal segments, hence its name *dens angularis*. Here it is subjected to lateral and protrusive forces which would readily loosen it were it not for its firm anchorage by means of its long, massive root, creating a prominent bulge in the bony alveolus enveloping it. This is called the canine eminence and is important in the determination of a normal facial profile.

The canine possesses some of the features of both the incisors and the premolars. The central lobe of the incisive edge is elongated to form a single pointed cusp with a mesial and distal slope, and the cingulum is much more pronounced than in the incisors, but not to the extent of developing into a palatal cusp, as in the premolars. It is the strongest tooth in the mouth, although it has undergone considerable reduction during man's phylogenic development. The crown is not excessively long and is compatible with the human temporomandibular joint in allowing lateral excursive movements in the mastication of an omnivorous diet. This is not the case with carnivores and anthropoid apes, where the length of the canine permits only a simple, vertical, chopping movement of the mandible.

The Premolars

There are two premolars on either side of the dental arch, named 'first' and 'second' from the midline and are unique to the permanent dentition. They replace the deciduous molars, and are also known as 'bicuspids' because they usually have two cusps, one buccal, one lingual. Their function is intermediate between that of the canines and the molars through their position in the jaw. The first premolars are adjacent to the canines and have an elongated buccal cusp so that from the buccal aspect they resemble the canine. This would indicate that they share its function in tearing food. Farther posteriorly, the second premolars are situated adjacent to the molars and have a crown form adapted more for the function of crushing. The buccal cusp, although larger, is rounded and less pronounced, whereas the occlusal surface is more obvious. The crown is much smaller than that of the molars, however, with a completely different morphology. The premolars have a single root except for the maxillary first premolar which has a buccal and palatal root.

The mandibular first premolar is smaller than the second, the opposite arrangement exists between the maxillary premolars.

The crowns of mandibular premolars have a marked lingual inclination whereas those of the upper premolars are placed centrally on the root.

The Permanent Molars

The permanent molars are the most posteriorly situated teeth in the mouth, and are named 'first', 'second' and 'third' according to their position from the midline. They do not replace any deciduous teeth.

The molars have the largest occlusal surfaces of all the teeth and have the important masticatory function of crushing and grinding food. They have anything from three to five main cusps, and are the only teeth with more than one buccal cusp. Between the cusps are complex groove, ridge and fissure patterns characteristics for each tooth and these are detailed in the individual descriptions of the various teeth.

Strong, divergent roots provide the molars with the necessary firm anchorage in the jaws for the heavy grinding function of these teeth. The mandibular molars have two roots, one mesial and one distal; the maxillary molars have three roots, mesiobuccal, distobuccal and palatal, of which the palatal is the largest.

Generally speaking, the outlines and contours of the maxillary molars are similar. There are usually four cusps, the distolingual being the smallest, and they are more pronounced than those of the permanent mandibular molars. The first maxillary molar is larger than the second, which is in turn larger than the third, and this is mainly due to a gradual reduction in size of the distolingual cusp, which may even be absent in third molars. The occlusal outline of maxillary molars is rhomboidal compared with the more oblong outline of mandibular molars. The buccal and lingual sides of the rhomboid are parallel with the curve of the dental arch. The proximal surfaces are in line with imaginary lines radiating outwards from a point in the midline of the posterior edge of the hard palate. The crowns of the maxillary molars are seated centrally on the roots whereas those of the mandibular molars incline lingually, a characteristic of all posterior mandibular teeth.

The mandibular molars have a rectangular or square occlusal outline. They have their widest measurement mediodistally in comparison with the upper molars which have a wider buccopalatal measurement. The first mandibular molar is the largest molar in the lower jaw. The third molar varies in size, however, and may be larger or smaller in comparison with the mandibular second molar. The roots of mandibular molars tend to curve distally.

Permanent Maxillary Dental Arch

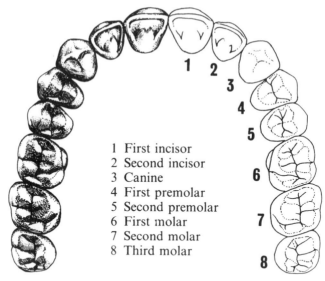

1 First incisor
2 Second incisor
3 Canine
4 First premolar
5 Second premolar
6 First molar
7 Second molar
8 Third molar

Fig. 29.

Permanent Mandibular Dental Arch

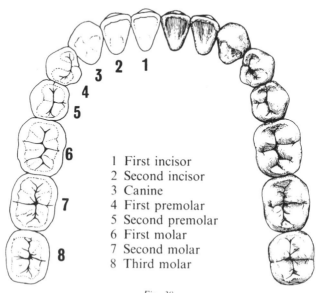

1 First incisor
2 Second incisor
3 Canine
4 First premolar
5 Second premolar
6 First molar
7 Second molar
8 Third molar

Fig. 30.

Maxillary First Permanent Incisor

Chronology

Initial calcification: 3–4 months after birth.
Completion of crown: 4–5 years.
Eruption: 7–8 years.
Completion of root: 10 years.

General

These teeth are often referred to as 'upper centrals' because they occupy the central space on either side of the midline of the maxilla. They are the largest of all the incisors although sometimes a maxillary lateral incisor may appear to be slightly longer overall. The crown is greater in bulk, however, being wider labiopalatally than the maxillary lateral incisor, and wider mesiodistally than any of the anterior teeth.

The labial surface of the crown is smooth, convex, and marked by two faint developmental grooves running vertically, which divide it into three lobes, giving the incisive edge in the unworn tooth three rounded protuberances called 'mamelons'.

The palatal surface of the crown is concave except for the pronounced convex cingulum, and confluent with this are the mesial and distal marginal ridges which extend to the incisive edge, enclosing the concave part of the crown, the *fossa linguale*.

The mesial and distal aspects give similar views showing the wedge-shaped crown with a solid base at the sinuous cervical margin and a thin incisive edge. Because the mesio-incisal angle is sharper than the disto-incisal, the mesial surface of the crown appears to be longer than the distal surface. The cervical margin of the crown·extends further incisally on the mesial side than on the distal side.

Generally, this is a very easy tooth to identify, and the only teeth with which it is sometimes confused are unusual variants of the maxillary lateral incisor.

Principal Identifying Features

1. *Mesial surface straight and at a sharp right-angle to incisive edge.*
2. *Disto-incisal angle more rounded.*
3. Crown large in proportion to root—widest anterior tooth.
4. Well-marked marginal ridges on concave palatal surface, with well-developed cingulum.
5. Crown inclined palatally; root inclined slightly distally.
6. Smooth, convex labial surface.
7. Cervical margin most sinuous on mesial side.
8. Single tapering root with rounded triangular cross-section, and one of the slightly flattened surfaces facing labially.

Variations

Malformed macrodont forms occasionally occur.

Exaggerated marginal ridges produce a shovel-shaped incisor form. This occurs more commonly in American Indian, Eskimo, Chinese and Japanese races.

The cingulum may be considerably elongated towards the incisive edge. A rare, and extreme form of this is the 'T-shaped incisor', resulting in an incisive edge shaped rather like the Mercedes symbol, when viewed from the incisal aspect.

i_1 superior, *see* page 15.

Endodontic anatomy, *see* page 109.

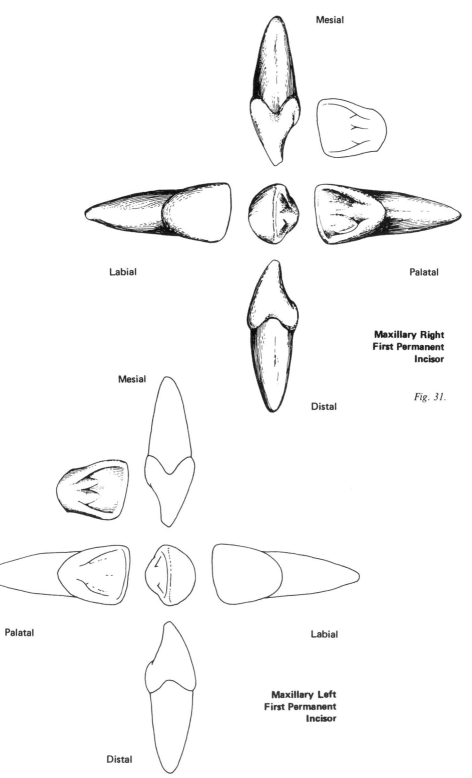

Mesial

Labial

Palatal

**Maxillary Right
First Permanent
Incisor**

Fig. 31.

Distal

Mesial

Palatal

Labial

**Maxillary Left
First Permanent
Incisor**

Distal

Fig. 32.

51

Mandibular First Permanent Incisor

Chronology

Initial calcification: 3–4 months after birth.
Completion of crown 4–5 years.
Eruption: 6–7 years.
Completion of root: 9 years.

General

The mandibular central incisors are the smallest of the permanent teeth and they occupy the central space on either side of the midline of the mandible.

The crown has the characteristic incisor form but is of diminutive proportions compared with the opposing maxillary central incisor.

The incisive edge has three small mamelons in the newly-erupted tooth. These soon become worn away so that most specimens of extracted mandibular central incisors have a straight incisive edge which is approximately at right-angles to the mesial and distal surfaces. The sharp mesio- and disto-incisal angles are best seen from the labial or lingual aspect.

The crown inclines more lingually than in the maxillary incisors, and from the incisal aspect the incisive edge can be seen to be on the lingual side of the central axis of the tooth, and if a line were to bisect the tooth labiolingually it would be at right-angles to it.

The lingual surface, unlike that of the maxillary central incisor, is relatively smooth and featureless with the marginal ridges and the cingulum being less well developed. The incisive and middle thirds show a shallow concavity, and towards the cervical third the lingual surface is convex because of a small cingulum.

The labial surface tends to be convex, particularly in the cervical third, and flattens out towards the incisive third.

This tooth has a single root which has approximately the same dimensions, labiolingually and longitudinally as that of the maxillary central incisor, but it is much thinner mesiodistally with a blunt apex.

Because of the symmetrical crown it is difficult to tell a left central incisor from a right, but the root may give three important clues: the mesial and distal surfaces both have a groove along their length, but that on the distal surface is more marked; the root tends to curve distally; and the cervical margin extends further incisally on the mesial side.

The mandibular central incisor is easily confused with the mandibular lateral incisor, and a comparison of both is essential.

Principal Identifying Features

1. *Single root, flattened mesiodistally, tends to curve distally.*
2. *Incisive edge at right-angles to a line bisecting crown labiolingually.*
3. Root 12 mm long.

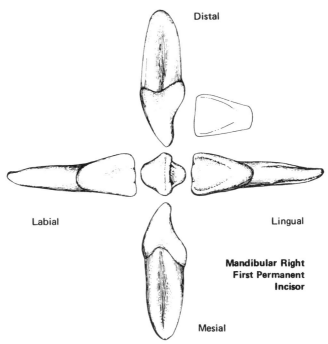

Distal

Labial

Lingual

Mandibular Right
First Permanent
Incisor

Mesial

Fig. 33.

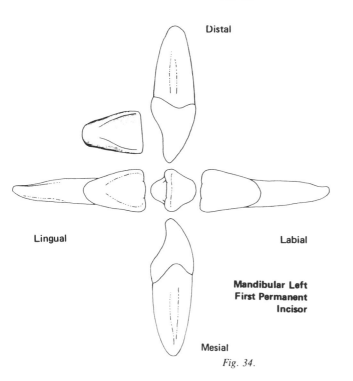

Distal

Lingual

Labial

Mandibular Left
First Permanent
Incisor

Mesial

Fig. 34.

4. Distal longitudinal groove on root more marked than mesial.
5. Smallest tooth in permanent dentition.

Variations

Sometimes two root canals present, one buccal, one lingual.
Rarely, root may be slightly bifurcated at apex.
Size of root or crown may vary.

i₁ inferior, *see* page 18.
I₂ inferior, *see* page 58.
Endodontic anatomy, *see* page 109.

Maxillary Second Permanent Incisor

Chronology

Initial calcification: 10–12 months after birth.
Completion of crown: 4–5 years.
Eruption: 8–9 years.
Completion of root: 11 years.

General

This tooth is second from the midline in the maxilla. The crown of the maxillary lateral incisor is blade-like, similar to that of the maxillary central incisor and has a wedge-shaped outline when viewed from the mesial or distal aspects. This fundamental incisor form enables it to supplement the function of the central incisors in the cutting or incising of food.

The general form of the crown closely resembles that of the maxillary central incisor although it is shorter and much narrower. The incisive edge shares the same characteristics in that the disto-incisal angle is more rounded and obtuse compared with the sharper mesio-incisal angle. These features are, however, exaggerated in the maxillary lateral incisor despite the fact that the crown is rounder overall.

The cingulum is visible from the palatal aspect, and is less pronounced than that of the central incisor. The palatal surface of the crown is concave, and sometimes to the extent of producing a deep shovel-shaped concavity, the *fossa linguale*. This is bordered mesially and distally by pronounced marginal ridges which fold together around the cingulum, ending in a pit of varying depth, the *foramen caecum incisivum*. Pathological extremes of this groove sometimes occur, resulting in an abnormally deep palatal pit, *dens invaginatus*, and this is prone to dental caries.

The maxillary second incisor is often difficult to identify because of these, and other extreme variations in its form (*see* 'Variations').

The single root is, in comparison with that of the maxillary central incisor, slightly longer in proportion to the crown. It is essentially round in cross-section and slightly flattened and grooved on the mesial and distal surfaces, tapering elegantly to a distally inclined apex.

Principal Identifying Features

1. *Mesio-incisal angle acute; disto-incisal angle more rounded.*
2. *Incisive edge has marked downward slope to the shorter distal surface.*
3. Crown more rounded, shorter, and narrower mesiodistally than maxillary central incisor.
4. Cingulum on palatal surface often encloses a pit, the *foramen caecum incisivum*.
5. Palatal surface more concave than that of maxillary central incisor.
6. Single root with elegant taper to pointed, distally-curving apex.
7. Cervical margin more sinuous on mesial surface than distal surface.

Variations

Subject to an enormous degree of variation, one common type being the peg-shaped lateral incisor which has a thin root surmounted by a small conical crown. Sometimes the crown is underdeveloped, bending sharply mesially. In approximately 5 per cent of cases, the *foramen caecum incisivum* is abnormally deep, resulting in a caries-prone invagination of the enamel on the palatal surface of the crown.

i_2 superior, *see* page 20.
I_1 superior, *see* page 49.
Endodontic anatomy, *see* page 110.

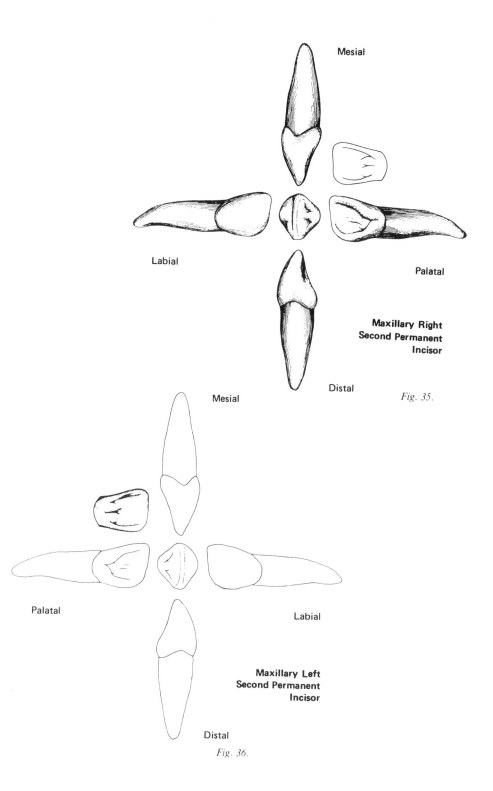

Mesial

Labial

Palatal

**Maxillary Right
Second Permanent
Incisor**

Distal

Fig. 35.

Mesial

Palatal

Labial

**Maxillary Left
Second Permanent
Incisor**

Distal

Fig. 36.

Mandibular Second Permanent Incisor

Chronology

Initial calcification: 3–4 months after birth.
Completion of crown: 4–5 years.
Eruption: 7–8 years.
Completion of root: 10 years.

General

The mandibular lateral incisor is situated second from the midline of the mandible, and is very similar to the mandibular central incisor.

In newly-erupted and unworn specimens three mamelons are seen on the incisive edge, which is slightly wider mesiodistally than that of the mandibular central incisor. The mesiodistal diameter of the cervices of both these teeth are, however, approximately the same, and hence the wider incisive edge of the mandibular lateral incisor gives this tooth a more fan-shaped appearance from the labial aspect.

This view also shows the mesial side of the crown to be slightly longer than the distal. The disto-incisal angle is relatively more rounded and obtuse than the sharp mesio-incisal angle.

Because the mandibular incisors resemble each other so closely, this is the one case where it is useful to refer to a tooth measurement to assist in identification. A comparison of the root lengths shows that when a measurement is taken from the lowest point of the anatomical crown to the root apex, the length of the root of the mandibular lateral incisor is, on average, 14 mm; that of the mandibular central incisor is shorter, approximately 12 mm.

The mesial and distal aspects of the two teeth are similar. They show the wedge-shaped crown with a solid base, of a similar labiolingual diameter to that of the mandibular central incisor, at the cervical margin, and a thin incisive edge.

Both teeth have a longitudinal groove on the mesial and distal surfaces of the roots, with the distal groove being more pronounced. The single root of the mandibular lateral incisor also tends to incline distally.

Perhaps the most important distinguishing feature is that the crown of the mandibular lateral incisor appears slightly askew on its root in order to allow the incisive edge to follow the curve of the dental arch. This means that from the incisal aspect, a line bisecting the root labiolingually would not be at right-angles to the incisive edge.

Principal Identifying Features

1. *Slightly larger than mandibular first incisor; fan-shaped crown, incisive edge wider mesiodistally.*
2. *Incisal aspect: incisive edge not at right-angles to bisecting line of root, but twisted distally in a lingual direction to follow line of dental arch.*

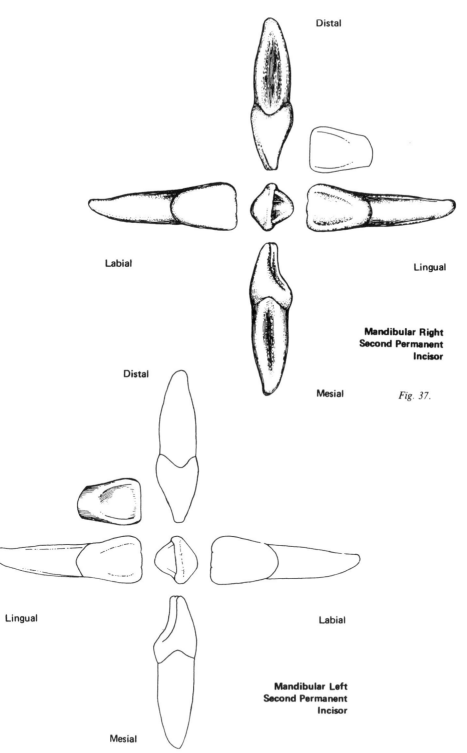

Distal

Labial

Lingual

**Mandibular Right
Second Permanent
Incisor**

Mesial

Fig. 37.

Distal

Lingual

Labial

Mesial

**Mandibular Left
Second Permanent
Incisor**

Fig. 38.

3. Root 14 mm long.
4. Mesial surface of crown slightly longer than distal so that incisive edge slopes slightly.
5. Faint mesial and distal marginal ridges but more pronounced than in mandibular first incisor.

Variations

No noticeable variations except for occasional differences in crown and/or root sizes.

i_2 inferior, *see* page 22.
I_1 inferior, *see* page 52.
Endodontic anatomy, *see* page 111.

Maxillary Permanent Canine

Chronology

Initial calcification: 4–5 months after birth.
Completion of crown: 6–7 years.
Eruption: 11–12 years.
Completion of root: 13–15 years.

General

The maxillary canine is the third tooth from the midline and is the longest tooth in the mouth by virtue of its strongly-developed single root which has similar contours to that of the maxillary central incisor.

The crown is very stout in character and convex on all surfaces, making its morphology radically different from that of the adjacent incisors. Its greater bulk of dentine, which gives it its strength, often gives the crown a slightly darker, more yellow appearance than the other teeth. The convex and relatively featureless surfaces also give the canine a certain amount of protection against decay.

There are two sites, however, which could be prone to decay, and these are the two shallow hollows which sometimes occur on the palatal surface between the bulky cingulum and the marginal ridges. These are the mesial and distal palatal fossae.

The incisive edge of the canine is surmounted by a large pointed cusp, with its tip placed approximately centrally, in line with the long axis of the tooth. It has a mesial and distal slope, the distal slope being longer. This is a primary clue when deciding to which side of the maxilla the tooth belongs, and is most clearly seen from the labial aspect. The smooth labial surface has a distinct convexity cervico-incisally. This is best viewed from the mesial and distal aspects, from which a number of other important features can also be seen. One point to notice is the profile of the large cingulum filling what would otherwise be a concave palatal surface. The cingulum also adds greatly to the labiopalatal measurement giving the maxillary canine the greatest circumference of all the anterior teeth.

The maxillary canine is an easy tooth to identify, and can only be confused with mandibular canines, especially when the specimen is old and worn.

Principal Identifying Features

1. *Single, pointed cusp approximately in line with long axis of root.*
2. *Distal slope of cusp longer than mesial slope, and confluent with convex distal surface.*
3. *Long stout proportions overall.*
4. Marked convex labial outline, and a bulky palatal cingulum.
5. Cervical line less sinuous on distal surface.
6. Very long single root with rounded triangular cross-section.
7. Disto- and mesiopalatal surfaces of root often grooved longitudinally.

Variations

Labiopalatal measurement may be exaggerated. Very occasionally, a supplementary cusp of variable size may be present on the distal slope of the incisive edge. Cingulum may be pointed (premolarization).
Tip of root sometimes bent sharply distally.

c superior, *see* page 24.
C inferior, *see* page 64.
Endodontic anatomy, *see* page 112.

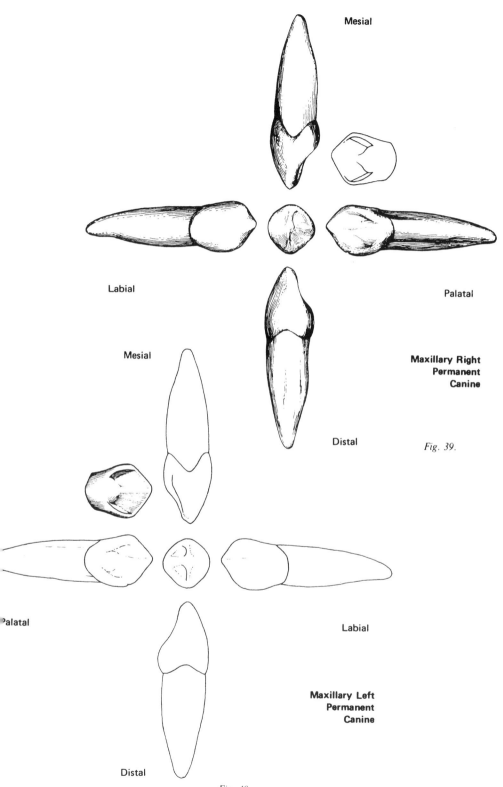

Mesial

Labial

Palatal

Mesial

Distal

**Maxillary Right
Permanent
Canine**

Fig. 39.

Palatal

Labial

**Maxillary Left
Permanent
Canine**

Distal

Fig. 40.

63

Mandibular Permanent Canine

Chronology

Initial calcification: 4–5 months after birth.
Completion of crown: 6–7 years.
Eruption: 9–10 years.
Completion of root: 12–14 years.

General

This is the third tooth from the midline of the mandible, and, although it is generally smaller and narrower than the maxillary permanent canine, the two teeth are sometimes confused because of their close resemblance. For this reason it is advisable to compare these teeth rather than try to study them individually.

Just as the features of the mandibular incisors are underdeveloped compared with their maxillary counterparts, the mandibular canine is less well developed than the upper. The marginal ridges and the cingulum are scarcely discernible, and the single cusp is less pointed than that of the maxillary canine, but is much narrower mesiodistally, which gives it the appearance of being longer. The labiolingual diameter of the crown at the cervical margin is also smaller than that of the maxillary canine.

The lingual surface of the crown is smooth, with a faint ridge running from the cusp tip to, and confluent with, the cingulum. On either side of this are two shallow hollows: the mesial and distal lingual fossae.

From the labial aspect, several important features of this tooth can be seen which not only identify it as the mandibular canine, but which also indicate to which side of the mandible it belongs: the crown appears to tilt distally on the root because its mesial surface is in approximately a straight line and continuous with the mesial surface of the root, and also because the distal outline is convex on the incisal half and concave on the cervical half; the mesial outline is longer and straighter than the distal; the mesial slope of the cusp is shorter than the distal, as in the maxillary canine, but the features are more rounded.

The labial aspect of the crown is convex and from the mesial or distal aspects its convex profile can be seen to be continuous with the vertical convexity of the long, solid root, so that together they form a gentle arc.

The mandibular permanent canine has a strong single root with an oval cross-section, being flattened and slightly grooved longitudinally on the mesial and distal surfaces. In a few cases the root may be seen to be partially bifurcated.

Principal Identifying Features

1. *Distal profile of crown more rounded than mesial.*
2. *Crown narrower mesiodistally than maxillary canine so that crown appears larger in proportion.*
3. Only the *mandibular* canine is capable of bifurcated root, a not uncommon variation.

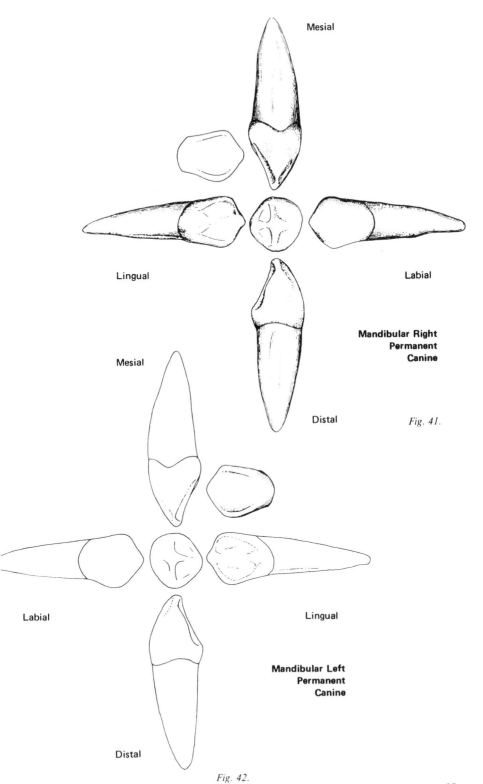

Mesial

Lingual

Labial

Mandibular Right Permanent Canine

Mesial

Distal

Fig. 41.

Labial

Lingual

Mandibular Left Permanent Canine

Distal

Fig. 42.

4. *Mesial slope of cusp shorter than distal.*
5. Poorly defined cingulum in comparison with upper canine.
6. Mesial surface of crown in approximately straight line with root.
7. Labial surface of crown in continuous longitudinal arc with root.
8. In most cases, root tends to curve slightly distally. Crown appears to lean distally in relation to root.

Variations

Single longitudinally-grooved root with *two* root canals.
Partial bifurcation of root to a labial and a lingual root.
Size of root and/or crown may vary.

c inferior, *see* page 27.
C superior, *see* page 61.
Endodontic anatomy, *see* page 113.

Maxillary First Premolar

Chronology

Initial calcification: 18–21 months after birth.
Completion of crown: 5–6 years.
Eruption: 10–11 years.
Completion of roots: 12–13 years.

General

The maxillary first premolar is the fourth tooth from the midline of the maxilla. Its function, along with the second premolar, is to crush food and divide it into smaller pieces.

From the buccal aspect, the crown resembles that of the maxillary canine, except that the mesial slope is longer than the distal slope. This arrangement is reversed in the maxillary canine.

The maxillary first premolar has a distinct depression on its mesial surface, extending from the cervical half of the crown to the root bifurcation. This is the *fossa canina*, mesial developmental depression, or canine fossa, and it is generally assumed that it is caused by pressure from the bulky and earlier completed crown of the maxillary first canine. It is not certain if this is the correct explanation for the formation of the canine fossa, but it is in any case an easy way of committing this important morphological feature to memory. If a single root is present, the concavity is very obvious.

Although, generally, this is the only premolar with two roots, this must be regarded only as a secondary identifying feature since the maxillary second premolars may occasionally have double roots, but then of course, no canine fossa.

The cusps of the maxillary first premolar are sharper than those of the maxillary second premolar. The palatal cusp is somewhat smaller than the buccal cusp, with its tip placed just mesially to the buccopalatal centre line of the crown. From the occlusal aspect, the crown appears more angular than that of the maxillary second premolar, being wider on its buccal side than on its palatal side. The two cusps are separated by a deep mesiodistal developmental fissure, which crosses over the mesial marginal ridge to merge into the concave mesial surface.

Principal Identifying Features

1. *Two roots, buccal and palatal—tend to curve distally.*
2. *Two sharply-defined cusps: buccal larger than palatal.*
3. *Concave canine fossa on mesial surface of crown extending to pronounced longitudinal groove on mesial surface of root.*
4. *Central developmental groove interrupts mesial marginal ridge.*
5. *Mesial slope of buccal cusp longer than distal.*
6. *Palatal cusp tilts slightly mesially.*
7. *Occlusal outline more angular than the maxillary second premolar.*

Variations

Variations are present mainly in the root: the buccal root may be divided into a mesio- and distobuccal root giving a total of three roots (and three root canals) or there may be just a single, longitudinally-grooved root. The roots can vary in form from short and blunt, to long and slender.

P_2 superior, *see* page 73.
Endodontic anatomy, *see* page 113.

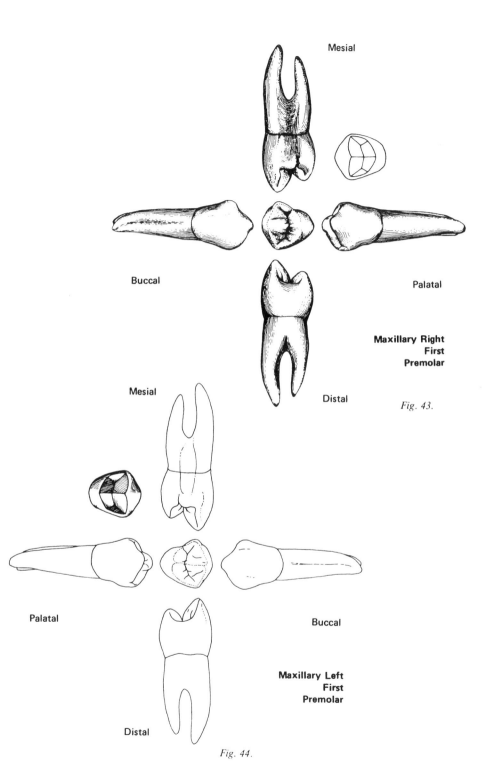

Mesial

Buccal

Palatal

**Maxillary Right
First
Premolar**

Mesial

Distal

Fig. 43.

Palatal

Buccal

**Maxillary Left
First
Premolar**

Distal

Fig. 44.

69

Mandibular First Premolar

Chronology

Initial calcification: $1\frac{3}{4}$–2 years.
Completion of crown: 5–6 years.
Eruption: 10–12 years.
Completion of root: 12–13 years.

General

The mandibular first premolar is situated fourth from the midline of the mandible, and is smaller than the mandibular second premolar; the opposite arrangement exists between the maxillary premolars.

It is also the smallest premolar in the human dentition, and has two cusps and an obvious premolar morphology, although it also possesses some of the characteristics of the neighbouring mandibular canine.

The buccal cusp is much larger than the lingual cusp, which in many cases is not high enough to occlude with the maxillary teeth. This causes the occlusal surface to slope approximately 45° lingually, and is best seen from the mesial or distal aspects. From this viewpoint, the lingual inclination of the crown is evident, a characteristic of all the posterior mandibular teeth. The tip of the buccal cusp is placed approximately centrally over the long axis of the root.

From the buccal aspect the mesial slope of the cusp is shorter than the distal, and the crown profile is therefore similar to that of the mandibular canine.

A number of important features may be seen from the occlusal aspect: the well-marked mesial and distal marginal ridges each enclose a fossa on either side of a ridge of enamel running from the large buccal cusp to the diminutive lingual cusp; the distal fossa is generally larger than the mesial fossa; the peripheral outline of the occlusal surface is approximately circular but flattened mesiolingually, as if by a chord, and this area accommodates the mesiolingual developmental groove.

The root is single, rounded, and usually curves distally, It is grooved longitudinally on the mesial and distal surfaces, with the mesial groove more marked, resembling the canine fossa of the maxillary first premolar.

Principal Identifying Features

1. *Two occlusal fossae, distal larger than mesial.*
2. *Two cusps joined by central enamel ridge: large pointed buccal cusp with centrally placed apex; diminutive lingual cusp.*
3. *Marked lingual inclination of crown on root.*
4. Buccal surface of crown convex; lingual surface almost straight.
5. Circular occlusal outline flattened and grooved on mesiolingual surface.
6. Single rounded root, tends to curve distally. Mesial longitudinal groove more marked than distal.

70

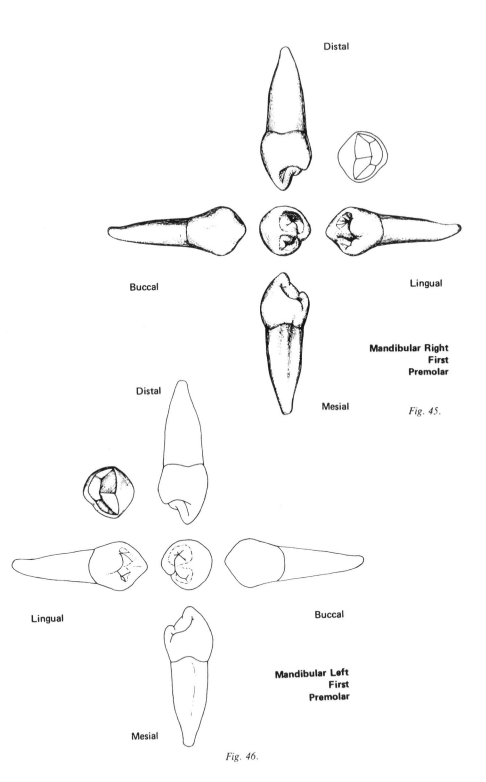

Distal

Buccal

Lingual

**Mandibular Right
First
Premolar**

Mesial

Fig. 45.

Distal

Lingual

Buccal

Mesial

**Mandibular Left
First
Premolar**

Fig. 46.

71

Variations

Lingual cusp may be larger than normal or, at the other extreme, it may be absent altogether, so that it resembles the cingulum of the mandibular canine. Accessory cusps may be present on the slopes of the buccal and lingual cusps. The root is bifurcated in rare cases.

Crown occasionally displays two lingual cusps, as in the second premolar.

P_2 inferior, *see* page 76.

Endodontic anatomy, *see* page 114.

Maxillary Second Premolar

Chronology

Initial calcification: 2–2½ years.
Completion of crown: 6–7 years.
Eruption: 10–12 years.
Completion of root: 12–14 years.

General

The maxillary second premolar is the fifth tooth from the midline of the maxilla, and resembles the maxillary first premolar in many ways, so that it is advisable to compare these two teeth rather than study them individually. There are, however, a few important differences: the maxillary second premolar is smaller with a more rounded crown; the mesiodistal developmental fissure does not interrupt the mesial marginal ridge; there is no canine fossa; the crown form is more symmetrical with both cusps centrally placed in relation to each other, and of equal height; the maxillary second premolar has, in nearly all cases, a single root.

The root is longer than both the roots of the maxillary first premolar, and the cusps are not as high which makes the crown appear shorter. These two factors make the proportions of crown to root considerably different between those two teeth.

From the buccal aspect, the buccal cusp of the maxillary second premolar shows a similar, but smaller and more rounded, outline to that of the maxillary canine. The distal slope of this cusp, like that of the canine, is longer than the mesial, and this is a useful guide in indicating the provenance of the tooth.

A pattern may be discerned in the maxillary premolars and the maxillary canine when they are considered from the buccal aspect. This makes the differences in the slopes of the buccal cusps easier to remember. In the maxillary canine, the maxillary first premolar and the maxillary second premolar the mesial slopes of the cusps are short, long, short, respectively. Similarly, the distal slopes are long, short, long.

Principal Identifying Features

1. *Two cusps, one palatal, one buccal: shallower and more equal in size than in maxillary first premolar.*
2. *No canine fossa—mesial surface convex.*
3. *Oval occlusal outline.*
4. *Single root flattened mesiodistally—longer than roots of maxillary first premolar.*
5. *Mesial slope of buccal cusp shorter than distal slope—exactly opposite to the situation in the maxillary first premolar but similar to the maxillary canine.*
6. *Occlusal mesiodistal fissure does not interrupt mesial marginal ridge. Tendency for additional fissures and grooves.*

Variations

Crown may flare out or taper in from the cervix. As in the maxillary canine, there may occasionally be an accessory cusp on the distal slope of the buccal cusp. Additional shallow grooves radiating from the central fissure may be present. Very rarely the root shows a tendency to bifurcate and follow the root form of the maxillary first premolar (not more than 10 per cent).

A rare variation in the crown form is the presence of three cusps. This is called molarisation. Apart from the two cusps which are normally present, namely the buccal (*paraconus*) and the palatal cusp (*protoconus*) there is a third cusp placed distopalatally (*hypoconus*).

P_1 superior, *see* page 67.
Endodontic anatomy, *see* page 115.

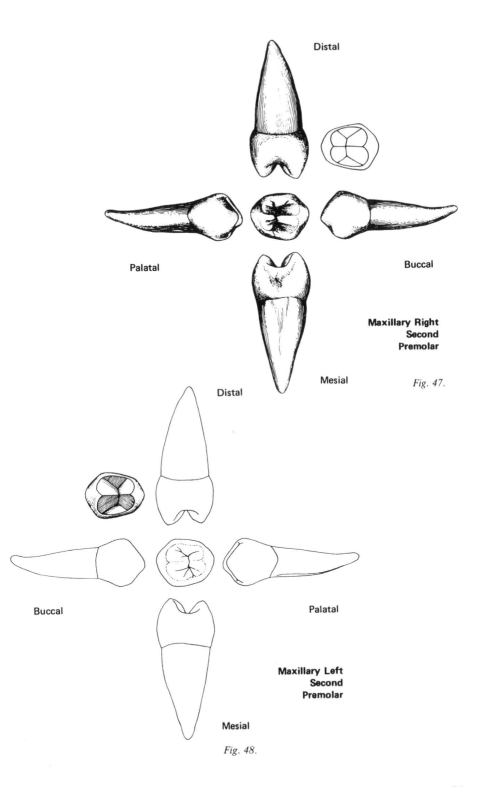

Distal

Palatal

Buccal

Mesial

**Maxillary Right
Second
Premolar**

Fig. 47.

Distal

Buccal

Palatal

Mesial

**Maxillary Left
Second
Premolar**

Fig. 48.

Mandibular Second Premolar

Chronology

Initial calcification: $2\frac{1}{4}$–$2\frac{1}{2}$ years.
Completion of crown: 6–7 years.
Eruption: 11–12 years.
Completion of root: 13–14 years.

General

This is the fifth tooth from the midline and the mandible, and supplements the function of the mandibular first premolar in crushing food. Unlike the maxillary premolars, however, there are obvious morphological differences: the mandibular second premolar is larger; has mostly three instead of two cusps; the lingual cusps are higher, resulting in a shallower lingual inclination of the occlusal surface (30° from the horizontal instead of 45°); the occlusal profile is more square instead of circular.

The occlusal morphology of the mandibular second premolar is variable with either two or three cusps. The illustration shows a three-cusped example because this form occurs most commonly. The variation occurs in the lingual cusp which, in both forms, is more pronounced than that of the lower first premolar. Either it may present as a single cusp, or it may be divided into two cusps giving a more angular, square outline, in which case the cusps are named as follows, in decreasing order of size and height: buccal cusp; mesiolingual cusp; distolingual cusp.

The buccal cusp is more rounded, shorter, and not quite so far placed over the long axis of the root as that of the mandibular first premolar, but it nevertheless makes up the bulk of the crown.

In the two-cusped form the buccal cusp is connected to the lingual cusp by a feint ridge of enamel confluent with both cusps. The mesial and distal fossae lie on either side of the ridge, and are bounded by the well-formed mesial and distal marginal ridges. As in the mandibular first premolar, the distal fossa is larger than the mesial fossa. The two fossae are connected by a central developmental groove which *curves* mesiodistally *around* the lingual side of the buccal cusp. When it reaches the enamel ridge connecting the two cusps it either runs over it or ploughs through it, making the ridge scarcely discernible. In the maxillary premolars the central developmental groove runs in practically a *straight* line because the cusps are more similar in size.

The three-cusped form of the mandibular second premolar presents a different occlusal pattern. The outline is more square and can, in some cases, be wider mesiodistally on the lingual side. There is a central pit with three grooves radiating from it: the mesial and distal developmental grooves running to the mesial and distal fossae respectively, and the lingual groove which extends between the two lingual cusps to the lingual surface.

Both mandibular premolars have a single root, but that of the mandibular second premolar tends to be slightly stouter and longer. It is more or less circular in cross-section and has a blunt conical apex which curves distally. Unlike the mandibular first premolar, there is no longitudinal grooving present on the root.

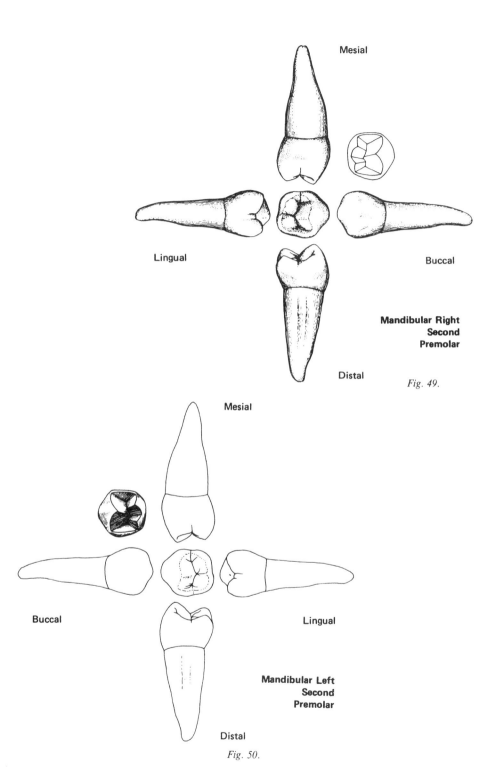

Mesial

Lingual

Buccal

Distal

**Mandibular Right
Second
Premolar**

Fig. 49.

Mesial

Buccal

Lingual

Distal

**Mandibular Left
Second
Premolar**

Fig. 50.

Principal Identifying Features

1. *Larger crown than mandibular first premolar.*
2. *Cusps more equal in size and less pointed, usually three cusps.*
3. Occlusal outline almost squarish with no mesiolingual flattening.
4. Central fissure *curves* around buccal cusp to join mesial and distal fossae; distal fossa larger.
5. Mesial marginal ridge higher than distal.
6. Single conical root, flattened slightly mesiodistally, curving distally to blunt apex.
7. No longitudinal grooves present.

Variations

Crown is subject to more variation than the mandibular first premolar. It may flare out to a wide occlusal surface from a narrow cervix, and may show two or three-cusped forms.

Very rarely, the root may be partially bifurcated.

P$_1$ inferior, *see* page 70.

Endodontic anatomy, *see* page 116.

Maxillary First Permanent Molar

Chronology

Initial calcification: Birth or slightly before.
Completion of crown: $2\frac{1}{2}$–3 years.
Eruption: 6–7 years.
Completion of roots: 9–10 years.

General

This is the largest tooth in the maxilla, and typifies the maxillary molar form in having a large crown with four major cusps and a wide occlusal surface, designed for grinding food. In approximately 50–70 per cent of cases, a fifth cusplet is present on the palatal surface of the mesiopalatal cusp. This is known as the cusp or tubercle of Carabelli and occurs usually bilaterally in the mouth. It can be easily felt by the tongue, but the degree to which it projects from the mesiopalatal cusp varies considerably, so that it is often so poorly formed as to be barely discernible, or so overdeveloped that it occupies the palatal surface between the mesio- and distopalatal cusps, thus deforming the occlusal surface by widening the mesial half of the crown.

The cusps are situated at the corners of the rhombic occlusal outline, and they are named according to their positions as follows (in decreasing order of size): mesiopalatal; mesiobuccal; distobuccal; cusp of Carabelli. Although the mesiopalatal cusp is the *largest*, the mesiobuccal cusp is the *highest*. The occlusal surface is widest diagonally from the mesiobuccal to the distopalatal cusp. The mesiopalatal and distobuccal angles are obtuse; the mesiobuccal and distopalatal angles are acute.

The four cusps are separated by a fissure pattern in the shape of an 'H'. The horizontal bar of the letter 'H' is formed by a fissure which crosses the oblique ridge (crista obliqua). The oblique ridge joins the mesiopalatal and distobuccal cusps. The maxillary first molar has three roots whose positions can easily be remembered by simple geometry: the buccal diameter of the maxilla is greater than the palatal diameter and can therefore accommodate more roots, and hence there are two buccal roots and one palatal. This applies to all maxillary molars. The palatal root is the longest and most divergent in order to follow the bone around the maxillary antrum. Both the buccal roots tend to curve distally. The distobuccal root is shorter than the mesiobuccal root.

The maxillary first permanent molar and the maxillary second deciduous molar resemble each other closely. A comparative study of these two teeth is advisable, especially since they are close neighbours in the mixed dentition from the age of six years, and may be confused with each other in clinical practice.

Principal Identifying Features

1. *Cusp of Carabelli on palatal surface of mesiopalatal cusp in 50–70 per cent of cases.*

2. Three well-developed and separated roots; palatal root longest and most divergent. Buccal roots tend to curve distally.
3. Rhomboidal occlusal outline.
4. Largest maxillary tooth.
5. Four cusps: mesiopalatal largest; distopalatal smallest; characteristic oblique ridge joining mesiopalatal and distobuccal cusps.
6. Buccal cusps more pointed than palatal cusps.
7. Crown wider buccolingually than mesiodistally.

Variations

The cusp of Carabelli is sometimes absent. Very occasionally, partial fusion of the buccal roots, or of the palatal and distobuccal root, may occur. A very rare variation is partial division of the palatal or mesiobuccal root.

Enamel pearls occasionally occur cervically on the mesial or distal surfaces. The distopalatal cusp (hypoconus) may sometimes be underdeveloped. Another rare variation is an extra small root on the buccal side, a so-called *radix paramolaris*, associated with the mesiobuccal root.

A shallow concavity may sometimes be present on the palatal surface of the palatal root, next to the cemento-enamel junction. This is a site of predilection for dental caries.

m$_1$ superior, *see* page 30.
m$_2$ superior, *see* page 36.
Endodontic anatomy, *see* page 117.

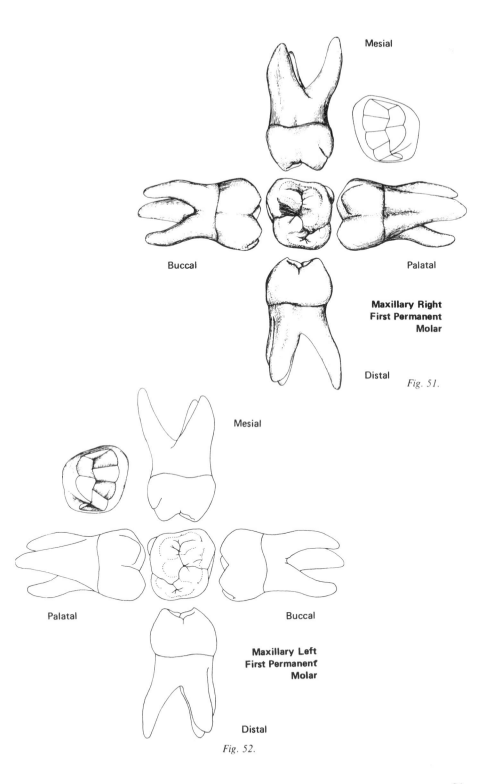

Mesial

Buccal

Palatal

**Maxillary Right
First Permanent
Molar**

Distal

Fig. 51.

Mesial

Palatal

Buccal

**Maxillary Left
First Permanent
Molar**

Distal

Fig. 52.

81

Mandibular First Permanent Molar

Chronology

Initial calcification: Birth or slightly before.
Completion of crown: $2\frac{1}{2}$–3 years.
Eruption: 6–7 years.
Completion of roots: 9–10 years.

General

The mandibular first permanent molar is situated sixth from the midline of the mandible, and is normally the largest mandibular tooth. It has five cusps, and these are, in decreasing order of *size*: mesiolingual, distolingual, mesiobuccal, distobuccal, distal. (The distal cusp is situated on the buccal side, distal to the distobuccal cusp.) In decreasing order of *height* the arrangement is different: mesiobuccal, mesiolingual, distobuccal, distolingual, distal.

In approximately 90 per cent of cases, the occlusal fissures display a *dryopithecus* pattern, so that instead of the cross-shaped fissure pattern, typical of mandibular molars, it is Y-shaped, formed by the lingual and the two buccal fissures, with the bases of the mesiolingual and distolingual meeting at the central fossa instead of the mesiobuccal and distolingual cusps. (It is important to remember that the distobuccal cusp is the second cusp on the buccal side, and not the third, which is called simply the distal cusp or *hypoconulus*.) The *dryopithecus* pattern is so called because it is present in all the lower molars of dryopithecine and anthropoid apes.

Because the buccal side accommodates an extra cusp, its mesiodistal measurement is longer than that of the lingual side. This is best seen from the occlusal aspect which shows a roughly oblong outline with the mesial and distal surfaces converging towards the lingual surface. The mesiodistal diameter is greater than the buccolingual, and this is characteristic of all the mandibular molars, unlike the maxillary molars in which the opposite proportions are found.

A helpful way of distinguishing this tooth from all the other molars is to hold the tooth upright and view it with one eye closed. From the buccal aspect all five cusps will be visible, but from the lingual aspect only three can be seen. This is because the more pointed lingual cusps obscure the slightly lower mesio- and distobuccal cusps, so that only the distal cusp and the two lingual cusps are visible.

The distal marginal ridge is not as tall as the mesial, and is often broken by a continuation of the central segmental groove which may extend onto the distal surface itself.

The buccal surface of the crown is markedly convex, and is divided into three lobes, each surmounted by one of the buccal cusps. Between these lobes runs a shallow groove, extending from the occlusal fissure between the mesio- and distobuccal cusps, and terminating in a buccal pit in approximately 60 per cent of cases. This is the *foramen caecum molarum*, and is a site of predilection for dental caries. Occasionally a second pit exists between the distobuccal and distal cusps. These pits are not always necessarily connected to the buccal fissures.

The mandibular first permanent molar has two roots that join at a common root trunk a few millimetres below the cervical margin. The mesial root is flat, with a

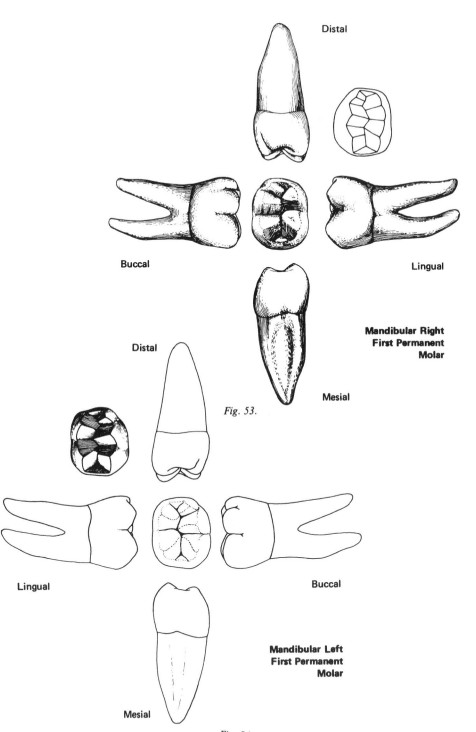

Distal

Buccal

Lingual

Mandibular Right First Permanent Molar

Distal

Mesial

Fig. 53.

Distal

Lingual

Buccal

Mandibular Left First Permanent Molar

Mesial

Fig. 54.

83

longitudinal groove on its mesial surface, and curves distally. The distal root is more rounded in cross-section and slightly shorter.

Principal Identifying Features

1. *Five cusps: three buccal, two lingual.*
2. *Bulbous, lingually-inclined buccal surface with two grooves.*
3. Largest mandibular tooth.
4. Buccal aspect: all five cusps visible.
   Lingual aspect; three cusps visible.
5. Crown longer mesiodistally than buccolingually; buccal surface longer than lingual.
6. Occlusal outline approximately oblong.
7. Primitive *dryopithecus* pattern present in nearly all cases, i.e. five-cusped tooth with bases of mesiolingual and centrobuccal cusps meeting at the central fossa.
8. Two roots: mesial root longer, flattened mesiodistally, grooved longitudinally and curved distally; distal root more rounded and less distally curved.

Variations

There may be four cusps instead of five as a result of reduction of the distal cusp (*hypoconulus*), giving a more circular outline similar to that of the mandibular second permanent molar.

Multi-apical variations: The mesial root may occasionally be partially bifurcated, giving the tooth three apices. The extra root is called the *radix paramolaris*. Another rare variation is the *radix entomolaris*, an accessory root growing out of the base of the distal root on the lingual side.

m_1 inferior, *see* page 33.
m_2 inferior, *see* page 39.
Endodontic anatomy, *see* page 118.

Maxillary Second Permanent Molar

Chronology

Initial calcification: $2\frac{1}{2}$–3 years.
Completion of crown: 7–8 years.
Eruption: 12–13 years.
Completion of roots: 14–16 years.

General

This tooth is the second molar and the seventh tooth from the midline of the maxilla and supplements the function of the maxillary first molar in crushing and grinding food.

Although the general form closely resembles that of the maxillary first permanent molar there are many features that enable it to be identified easily. The crown is generally smaller, with a much reduced distopalatal cusp (*hypoconus*) which may sometimes be absent altogether (*see* 'Variations').

The buccolingual diameter is approximately equivalent to that of the maxillary first molar, but the mesiodistal diameter is considerably less in proportion, which has the effect of emphasizing the rhomboidal outline of the maxillary second molar when viewed from the occlusal aspect. When the distolingual cusp is absent, the occlusal outline is more triangular, with a well-developed cusp at each corner. Care must be taken in identifying this latter type as it is a typical maxillary *third* molar form.

A cusp of Carabelli is not usually present in the maxillary second molar. The roots are approximately the same length as those of the maxillary first molar, but appear longer in proportion to the crown and tend to slope more distally. The palatal root is less divergent than and the two buccal roots are closer together than those of the maxillary first molar. This often results in coalescence, most commonly of the buccal roots, and also of one or both of them with the palatal root. Fusion of roots occurs more frequently in the maxillary second molar than the maxillary first molar (in approximately 30 per cent of cases).

In the maxillary first molar, the mesiobuccal root is more mesially placed than in the maxillary second molar where the apex of the mesiobuccal root lies more or less centrally above the buccal surface.

Principal Identifying Features

1. *No cusp of Carabelli.*
2. *Rhombic occlusal outline more obvious, and narrower mesiodistally than maxillary first molar.*
3. Roots less divergent; both buccal roots approximately the same length, closer together, parallel, slight distal inclination.
4. Coalescence of roots more common than in maxillary first molar.
5. Oblique ridge joins mesiopalatal and distobuccal cusps; both distal cusps greatly reduced in size.

85

6. Crown slightly smaller overall than maxillary first molar, although very close resemblance.

Variations

There are three main variations from the classic four-cusped form: (*a*) three cusps with the distolingual cusp absent; (*b*) three-cusped form compressed mesiodistally with the mesiobuccal, middle (coalescence of distobuccal and mesiolingual cusps), and the distolingual in a straight row; (*c*) similar to maxillary first molar crown morphology but with a reduced distolingual cusp.

Fusion of the roots sometimes occurs, especially between the two buccal roots or between the palatal and mesiobuccal roots.

The shape and size of the palatal root can vary.

Enamel pearls are occasionally present on the mesial or distal surfaces.

Very rarely, a cusp of Carabelli may be present.

m_2 superior, *see* page 36.
Endodontic anatomy, *see* page 119.

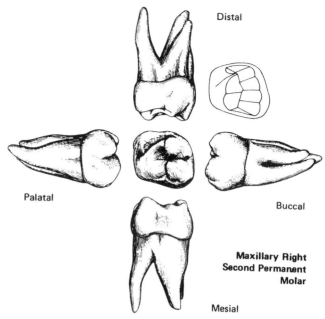

Distal

Palatal

Buccal

**Maxillary Right
Second Permanent
Molar**

Mesial

Fig. 55.

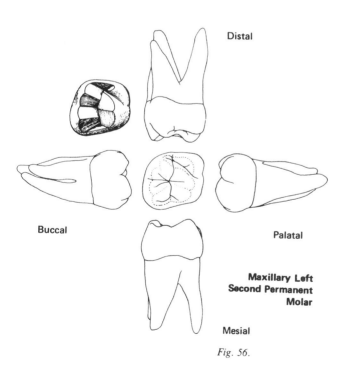

Distal

Buccal

Palatal

**Maxillary Left
Second Permanent
Molar**

Mesial

Fig. 56.

Mandibular Second Permanent Molar

Chronology

Initial calcification: $2\frac{1}{2}$–3 years.
Completion of crown: 7–8 years.
Eruption: 11–13 years.
Completion of roots: 14–15 years.

General

This is the seventh tooth from the midline of the mandible, and resembles the mandibular first molar in general form but has four cusps instead of five which as a result of the total reduction of the fifth distal cusp (*hypoconulus*) alters its occlusal profile and reduces its size.

This tooth has four cusps which are symmetrically situated at the rounded corners of the square peripheral outline of the occlusal surface with a cruciform groove pattern separating them. Think of this tooth as a hot-cross bun!

The two lingual cusps are higher than the two buccal cusps and are slightly more pointed. They are separated by the lingual groove which extends from the occlusal half of the lingual surface to the centre of the occlusal surface where it joins the buccal groove. The buccal groove separates the buccal cusps in a similar way and may terminate in a pit of the buccal surface. This pit is called the *foramen caecum molarum*, and is a site of predilection for dental caries.

The buccal surface of the crown is more convex and presents a larger surface area than the lingual surface. From the occlusal aspect, a good specimen shows a semicircular buccal outline, in contrast with the flat lingual outline, and much more of the buccal surface of the crown is visible than the lingual surface because of the lingual inclination of the crown.

The mesial and distal surfaces are similar although the distal surface may be slightly more convex. The two surfaces tend to converge from the buccal to the lingual, but this is scarcely discernible, and it is certainly not as marked as the convergence in the mandibular first molar. The mesial and distal aspects show the lingual inclination of the crown on the root, an important characteristic of all mandibular molars.

The mandibular second molar has two roots similar to the mandibular first molar, one mesial and one distal. They are closer together and curve more distally, with their axes approximately parallel compared with the more divergent roots of the mandibular first molar. Both roots are flattened mesiodistally and the mesial is larger.

It is advisable to compare this tooth with a specimen of a mandibular first permanent molar in order to appreciate more fully their individual features and differences.

Principal Identifying Features

1. *Rounded square occlusal outline.*

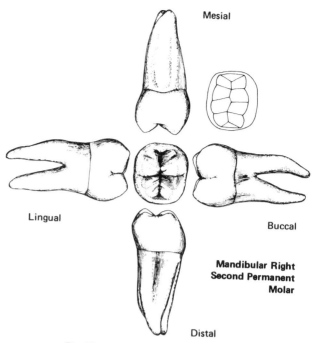

Mesial

Lingual

Buccal

**Mandibular Right
Second Permanent
Molar**

Distal

Fig. 57.

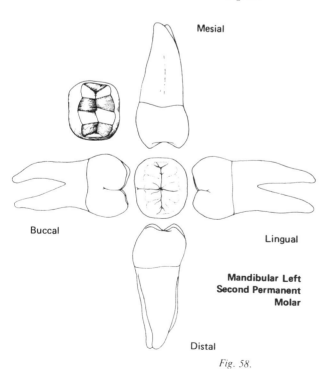

Mesial

Buccal

Lingual

**Mandibular Left
Second Permanent
Molar**

Distal

Fig. 58.

89

2. *Four cusps: two lingual, two buccal, separated by a pronounced central cruciform fissure pattern on occlusal surface.*
3. Not as wide mesiodistally as mandibular first molar.
4. Buccal surface bulbous and lingually inclined with one groove, terminating in a buccal pit, the *foramen caecum molarum.*
5. Lingual cusps higher than buccal cusps.
6. The mesial cusps are larger than the distal cusps.
7. Two roots similar to mandibular first molar but less broad, closer together and occasionally partially fused. Axes of both roots approximately parallel and curved distally.

Variations

May occasionally present a crown form similar to the mandibular first molar with three buccal and two lingual cusps.
Roots may sometimes be partially fused.
The distal curvature of the roots can vary greatly.
Very rarely, a *radix entomolaris* or partial division of the mesial root may be present. (A *radix entomolaris* is an accessory rootlet growing out of the lingual side of the base of the distal root.)

m$_2$ inferior, *see* page 39.
M$_1$ inferior, *see* page 82.
Endodontic anatomy, *see* page 119.

Maxillary Third Permanent Molar

Chronology

Initial calcification: 7–9 years.
Completion of crown: 12–16 years.
Eruption: 17–21 years.
Completion of roots: 18–25 years.

General

Normally speaking, this is the smallest maxillary molar and is situated farthest from the midline. It is known colloquially as the 'upper wisdom tooth' and varies to such a degree that this general description must be supplemented by a study of the 'Variations' section.

The typical crown form is similar to that of the maxillary second molar but it is not so well developed. The occlusal outline is roughly triangular because of the considerably reduced distopalatal cusp which is absent altogether in approximately 50 per cent of cases. When this cusp is absent there is no oblique ridge, but just a distal marginal ridge enclosing the distal side of a basic trigon.

As well as the crown, the roots are underdeveloped. They are usually three in number and their arrangement is similar to those of the other maxillary molars. They also tend to converge while sloping distally, and coalescence of two or three of these short roots to form an irregular conical mass is very common. Occasionally, additional vestigial roots are present.

There are three prominent cusps, and in many cases these are not very worn because the tooth has not been in functional occlusion. In some specimens, the occlusal surface has a wrinkled appearance because of additional grooves and fissures radiating from a deep central fossa.

This can be an easy tooth to identify, but, just as easily, it is possible to confuse it with the maxillary second molar. It is, therefore, often worth while scrutinizing the mesial surface, as any third molar should give evidence of one contact point only. This should not be thought of as a reliable guide, however, as there are many factors that can prevent the formation of a worn contact area.

Principal Identifying Features

1. *Triangular occlusal outline; diminutive distopalatal cusp often absent.*
2. *Roots short, underdeveloped, convergent, often fused, curve distally. Usually three in number.*
3. *Smallest maxillary molar*; crown smaller overall than maxillary second molar.
4. Largest cusp: mesiopalatal.
5. Mesial contact area only.
6. The crown often appears 'too big for its roots'!

Variations

The maxillary third molar is subject to more variation than any other tooth in the human dentition. Variants are usually smaller than other maxillary molars or sometimes so large and malformed as to be considered anomalous teeth. The crown may have a similar form to that of the maxillary second permanent molar, or may be underdeveloped and peg-shaped with a small tapering root.
Accessory cusps and roots may be present.
Extreme variations may occur in the degree of distal curvature of the roots.
Enamel pearls may occasionally be present.

M_2 superior, *see* page 85.
M_3 inferior, *see* page 94.
Endodontic anatomy, *see* page 120.

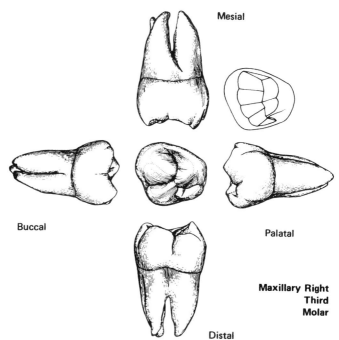

Mesial

Buccal

Palatal

Distal

**Maxillary Right
Third
Molar**

Fig. 59.

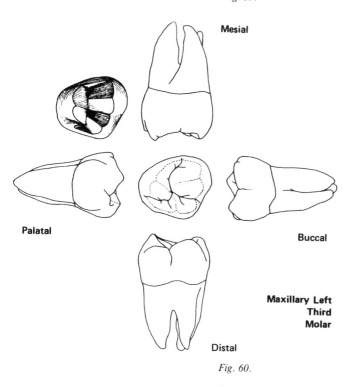

Mesial

Palatal

Buccal

Distal

**Maxillary Left
Third
Molar**

Fig. 60.

Mandibular Third Permanent Molar

Chronology

Initial calcification: 8–10 years.
Completion of crown: 12–16 years.
Eruption: 17–21 years.
Completion of roots: 18–25 years.

General

The mandibular wisdom tooth is the last tooth in the mandibular arch and is the eighth from the midline. It supplements the other mandibular molars in crushing and grinding food, although it is often prevented from fulfilling this function because of bad positioning, e.g. impaction. For this reason many specimens of third molars appear practically unworn.

A classic mandibular third molar has a crown form that is very similar to the mandibular second molar, with four cusps and a typical mandibular molar morphology as previously described, but with many more accessory fissures radiating from the central fossa. As in the maxillary wisdom tooth, this basic form is subject to a great deal of variation (*see* 'Variations'). The illustration shows a four-cusped form.

From the occlusal aspect, the marked convexity of the buccal surface is easy to distinguish from the flatter lingual surface. The peripheral occlusal outline, as a whole, is similar to the other mandibular molars in being roughly oblong or square, but the corners tend to be more rounded to the extent that some mandibular third molars have an almost circular occlusal outline. The bucco-lingual width of the tooth is smallest at the distal end.

The two roots, one mesial and one distal, are essentially similar to those of the other mandibular molars except that they are shorter and less well developed, or may tend to be fused together as one conical mass in some cases. The curvature of the roots is always distal, and usually more so than that of mandibular second molars. In the same way, the distal curvature of the roots of the mandibular second molar is more pronounced than that of the mandibular first molar. This indicates a progessive increase in the distal inclination of the roots as one moves further posteriorly.

No matter how many roots there may be to this tooth, it is nearly always possible to distinguish it from a maxillary third molar. The occlusal outline of mandibular molars is approximately oblong whereas the occlusal outline of maxillary molars is rhomboid. The crown of a mandibular molar is also lingually inclined in relation to its roots, whereas that of a maxillary molar is not.

Confusion of some specimens of mandibular third molars with other mandibular molars is possible, however, so that a comparative, rather than an individual, study of this tooth is advisable. A helpful clue, for worn cases, is that third molars can only show signs of interproximal wear on the mesial contact point.

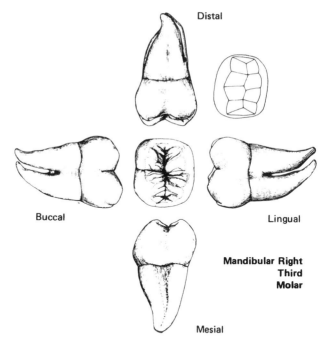

Distal

Buccal

Lingual

Mandibular Right
Third
Molar

Mesial

Fig. 61.

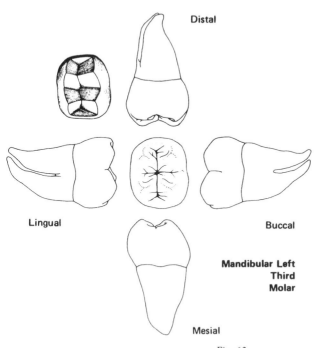

Distal

Lingual

Buccal

Mandibular Left
Third
Molar

Mesial

Fig. 62.

95

Principal Identifying Features

1. *Crown form similar to mandibular second molar, but mostly smaller.*
2. *Two roots: short, underdeveloped, often fused with a marked distal inclination.*
3. Square/oblong occlusal outline—corners well rounded.
4. Four cusps.
5. Buccolingual measurement least at distal end.
6. Markedly convex buccal surface inclined lingually.

Variations

A very variable tooth but less so than the upper wisdom teeth. Crown may show three, four, five or multi-cusped variations so that it is larger, in many cases, than the mandibular second molar, in which case it appears too big for its roots. The five-cusped variation resembles the mandibular first molar, but the under-developed and excessively distally curved roots indicate that the tooth in question is a third and not a first mandibular molar.

The occlusal surface may be very irregular with many accessory grooves radiating from a deep central fossa.

Multi-rooted forms sometimes occur.

A *radix entomolaris* may very occasionally be present (*see* M_1 and M_2 inferior).

M_2 inferior, *see* page 88.
M_3 superior, *see* page 91.
Endodontic anatomy, *see* page 121.

Section 3

Endodontic Anatomy

Introduction

All the teeth of the human dentition have a hollow space within them, containing the vital part of the tooth, the pulp or *pulpa dentis*. This hollow space can be divided into two main parts, the pulp chamber or *cavum dentis*, and root canal or *canalis radicis dentis*. The root canal extends from the pulp chamber to the root until it reaches the root apex or *apex radicis dentis*. Here the root canal terminates as a small opening, the apical foramen or *foramen apicis dentis*.

The pulp chamber of each tooth is simple in shape, and corresponds with the external shape of the tooth. A tooth with very pronounced cusps will also have a pulp chamber with the same number of pointed projections corresponding to each cusp. These projections of the pulp are called pulp horns or *cornua*, and are more obvious in young examples of teeth, than in old teeth. This is because secondary dentine is laid down with age. The laying down of secondary dentine against the walls of the entire pulp cavity results in a slow process of narrowing of the pulp chamber and root canals during the life of the tooth.

The root canals and the pulp chamber coincide, in most cases, at a point slightly apical to the cemento-enamel junction. This is also an area where accessory root canals may be present in molar teeth. These small, irregular canals connect the pulp directly with the blood vessel in the periodontium of the root furcation. These small canals are a result of incomplete filling-in of blood vessel canals during odontogenesis and the development of the tooth. These accessory canals are present in the apical part of the roots of all the teeth, and end around the surface of the root apex as accessory apical foramina or *foramina apicorum*, in an apical delta. Most of the accessory canals in dentine become calcified or considerably constricted with the laying down of secondary dentine. If they remain open, they can hinder the success of a normal orthograde root filling because they are very difficult to seal off completely.

The apical third of the root and the apical foramen together form a very important anatomical area as regards endodontic treatment. It consists of cement, the apical foramen, the apical constriction, and the apical delta, consisting of many small accessory canals (*see Fig. 63*).

The apical foramen is only sometimes to be found precisely in the middle of the root apex, and variations occur as a result of a curvature in the root canal at the apex. The apical foramen has in most cases, an extension of its entrance, made up of secondary cement, with the result that the original apical foramen lies 0·5–1·0 mm within the visible root apex. This difference increases with age as increasing amounts of secondary cement are laid down.

Approximately 0·5–1·0 mm before the true apical foramen lies the apical constriction, and the root canal is often narrower here than at the apical foramen. This is the point to which clinicians strive to seal off the root canal during endodontic treatment.

In order to study the pulp cavities of the teeth, it is advisable to split open a few examples. It goes without saying that the discovery of the pulp cavity *in vitro* is preferable now, than later *in vivo* during the course of the student's first experiences in clinical dentistry.

A selection should be made of young and old teeth, to include examples of each tooth type. They should then be split open carefully, but this is easier said than done, for teeth are not hazelnuts! The quickest way of doing this is with a diamond separating disc at high speed with water cooling. This is used to cut a groove in the tooth in the desired direction, before placing the tooth in a piece of Plasticine on a sturdy wooden block, with the groove facing upwards.

A sharp, 1-inch wood chisel is then applied to the groove, and a sharp but withdrawn blow is then given with a hammer.

This method of tooth cleaving gives reasonable results for simple studies of the pulp cavities of the teeth. There are, of course, much better methods available, such as acrylic resin injections of the pulp cavity, but they are too complicated, and unsuitable for superficial study of the pulp cavity.

The illustrations in this chapter on endodontic anatomy are based on the same technique used throughout the book, except that only three of the five elevations are shown in order to save space. The elevations chosen in each case are buccal, mesial and occlusal, with additional cross-sections through the tooth at the levels indicated by the broken lines on the buccal elevation.

The pulp cavities illustrated in this chapter are of young teeth and are therefore of maximum proportions.

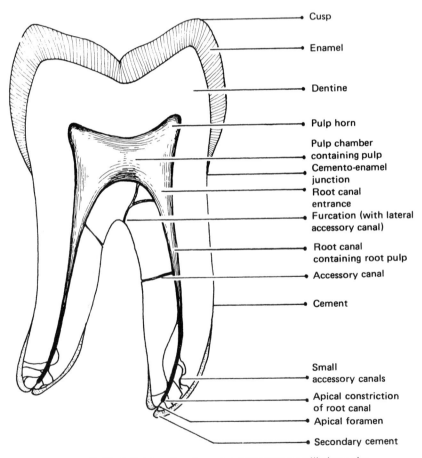

Cusp

Enamel

Dentine

Pulp horn

Pulp chamber containing pulp

Cemento-enamel junction

Root canal entrance

Furcation (with lateral accessory canal)

Root canal containing root pulp

Accessory canal

Cement

Small accessory canals

Apical constriction of root canal

Apical foramen

Secondary cement

Fig. 63. Mesiodistal section through a permanent mandibular molar.

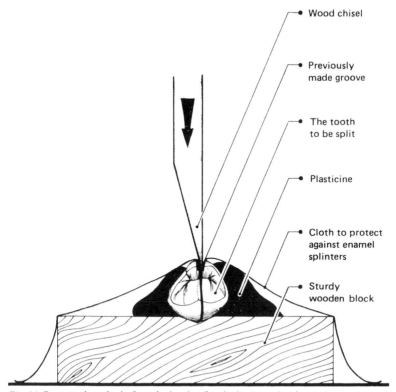

Wood chisel

Previously
made groove

The tooth
to be split

Plasticine

Cloth to protect
against enamel
splinters

Sturdy
wooden block

Fig. 64. Suggested method of tooth cleaving for the basic study of endodontic anatomy.

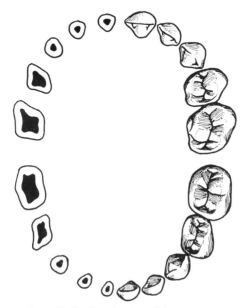

Fig. 65. Maxillary and mandibular dental arches of the deciduous dentition. On one side, the crowns of the teeth have been ground away at the level of the cemento-enamel junction in order to display the shapes of the pulp centres.

It is important to remember that a physiological deposition of secondary dentine occurs with age, resulting in a narrowing of the pulp chamber and the root canals. The pulp horns also become narrower, and sometimes lower in height.

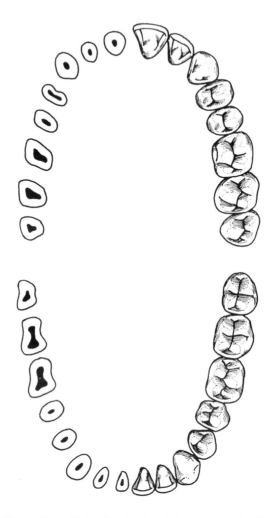

Fig. 66. Maxillary and mandibular dental arches of the permanent dentition. On one side, the crowns of the teeth have been ground away at the level of the cemento-enamel junction in order to display the shapes of the pulp cavities.

Endodontic Anatomy of the Deciduous Dentition

The anatomy of the deciduous teeth is not dealt with as fully as that of the permanent teeth for two reasons: first, the pulp cavities of the deciduous teeth are approximately similar to those of the corresponding permanent teeth, so that lengthy individual descriptions can be avoided by giving only a brief account of their principal differences; secondly, a thorough knowledge of the pulp anatomy of deciduous teeth is less important than in the permanent teeth, in order to perform a satisfactory endodontic treatment.

Because the pulp anatomy of the deciduous teeth is so similar in many cases, these teeth are described in groups, in contrast with the permanent teeth where the differing anatomical features necessitate individual descriptions.

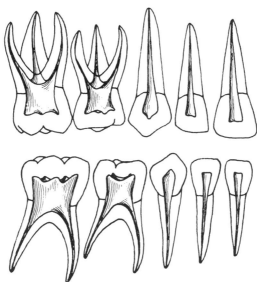

Fig. 67. Pulp cavities of the deciduous teeth.

General features of the pulp cavities of deciduous teeth

1. Smaller depth of dentine between the pulp chamber and the enamel, especially in the mandibular second deciduous molar.
2. Very thin, highly projecting pulp horns in the molars, especially mesial.
3. The pulp chamber is relatively larger than in the corresponding permanent tooth as a result of the thinner dentine walls which enclose it.
4. There are no clearly defined root canal entrances.
5. Long root canals; in the molars the root canals are often irregular and ribbon-like.
6. The root canals of the deciduous molars diverge greatly.
7. Thin enamel.

N.B. See also 'Principal Differences between Deciduous and Permanent Teeth', page 11.

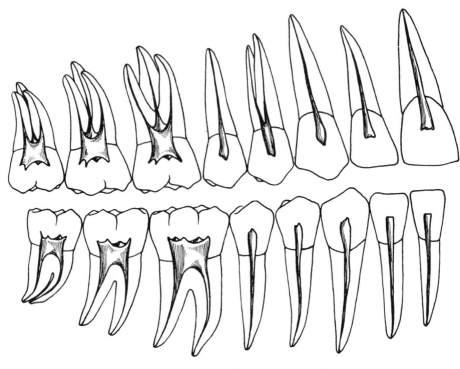

Fig. 68. Pulp cavities of the permanent teeth.

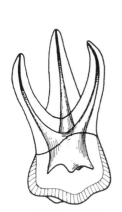

**Maxillary first
deciduous molar**

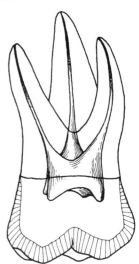

**Maxillary first
permanent molar**

Fig. 69. Comparison of a maxillary first *deciduous* molar with a maxillary first *permanent* molar. *N.B.* The deciduous tooth has a thinner layer of enamel covering the crown more evenly than that of the permanent tooth. The deciduous tooth has a relatively larger pulp cavity with longer pulp horns.

Deciduous incisor

The simple pulp chamber of this tooth is fan-shaped when viewed from the labial aspect, and corresponds with the shape of the crown. It is relatively wider than that of the permanent incisor and extends further incisally so that the pulp lies closer under the thin enamel covering the crown. Pulp exposures during even the most simple clinical cavity preparations occur quite frequently because of this.

The pulp horns are less pointed than in the permanent incisors. The pulp chamber is wedge-shaped labiolingually, and becomes narrower at the incisive edge.

The root canal is wide and splays out more than in the permanent incisors resulting in a relatively wider apical cross-section, without a clearly-defined apical

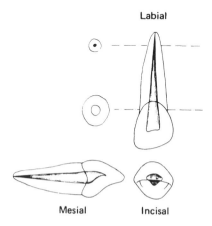

Fig. 70. Maxillary first incisor.

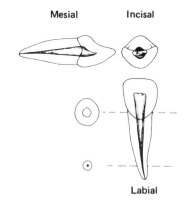

Fig. 71. Mandibular first incisor.

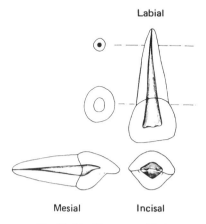

Fig. 72. Maxillary second incisor.

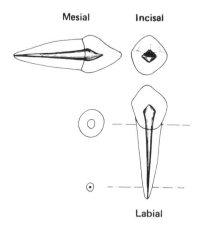

Fig. 73. Mandibular second incisor.

constriction. The root canal is widest labiolingually so that the mesiodistal flattening results occasionally in a partial division of the canal into two canals separated by a mesiodistal dentine dividing wall. In most cases, however, the deciduous incisors have only one root canal with an oval cross-section, ending in a relatively wide apical foramen. The apical third of the root is perforated by many accessory canals.

Deciduous canine

The pulp chamber of this tooth is similar in many ways to that of the deciduous incisors, except that it has a single pulp horn, corresponding with the external morphology of the crown.

There is no obvious morphological border between the pulp chamber and the root canal, so that the entire pulp cavity tapers evenly from the roof of the pulp chamber to the root apex, without being interrupted by constrictions.

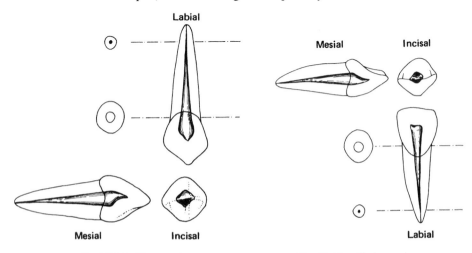

Fig. 74. Maxillary canine.

Fig. 75. Mandibular canine.

In cross-section, the root canal appears flattened on the mesial and distal sides giving it a slightly oval shape. The root canal of this tooth is longer than that of all the other deciduous teeth, and ends in an obvious apical foramen with many small accessory apical canals. The apical third tends to curve distally. The root canal is proportionally longer relative to the crown height, than in the permanent canines.

As is the case with all deciduous teeth, the dentine between the pulp chamber and the enamel layer covering the crown, is much less than in the permanent canine.

Deciduous molars

The pulp chamber of these teeth is very large relative to the external dimensions of the crown. This is especially true of the mandibular second molar. The dentine and enamel walls of these teeth are fairly thin, and the distance between the pulp horns and the enamel surface is sometimes as little as 2 mm. Special 'Eastman' burs are often advised for the preparation of cavities in deciduous molars in the hope of reducing the chances of pulp exposure during treatment.

The pulp chamber has the same number of pulp horns as there are cusps on the crown, and these extend quite far under the cusps. This is especially true of the mesial pulp horns, the most obvious example of which is present in the second molars.

The root canals are irregular, often ribbon-like and much more complicated than those in the permanent molars.

The root furcation is very close to the level of the cemento-enamel junction, so that lateral perforation is a risk at this point during endodontic treatment.

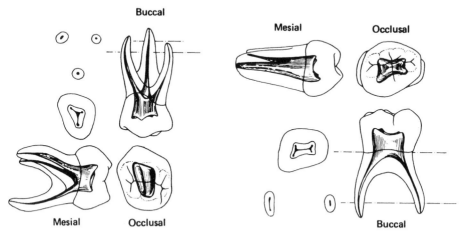

Fig. 76. Maxillary first molar.

Fig. 77. Mandibular first molar.

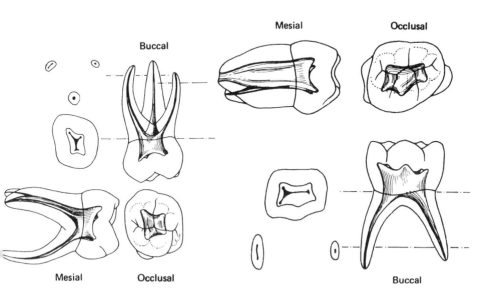

Fig. 78. Maxillary second molar.

Fig. 79. Mandibular second molar.

The maxillary molars have three roots, and often four root canals (two in the mesiobuccal root); the mandibular molars have two roots and four root canals (two in each root). The root canals diverge as strongly as the roots themselves, and often end as narrow apical splits, instead of round foramina, with many small accessory canals.

The roots of the molars are fully completed approximately two years after the eruption of the tooth.

Endodontic Anatomy of the Permanent Teeth

Maxillary first permanent incisor

This tooth has a simple pulp cavity, with a similar form to that of the maxillary second incisor. From a labial viewpoint, the pulp is fan-shaped, i.e. narrow at the cervix, spreading wider towards the incisive edge, where the pulp extends into a mesial and distal pulp horn. Young specimens have a third, central pulp horn, related to the central developmental lobe of the crown.

In the labiopalatal section, the pulp displays a wedge-shaped form becoming gradually narrower towards the incisive edge. Except in the rare instance of a pathological variation, this tooth has a single root canal, tapering gradually as it reaches the root apex. There is a slight constriction of this canal at the level of the root just apical to the cemento-enamel junction.

In cross-section, the root canal is oval in shape, becoming more circular in the apical third, and ending as a very narrow apical foramen at the apex.

Completion of *foramen apicale*: 10 years.

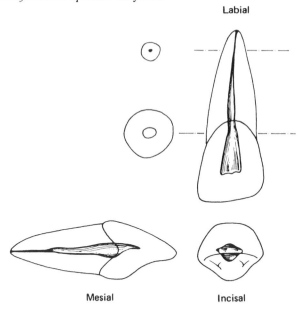

Labial

Mesial　　　**Incisal**

Fig. 80. Maxillary first permanent incisor.

Mandibular first permanent incisor

The shape of the pulp cavity of this tooth corresponds with that of the maxillary first incisor, but is smaller overall.

The shape of the pulp chamber is oval in cross-section, and flattened on the mesial and distal sides, compared with that of the maxillary first permanent incisor in which the labial and palatal sides are flattened.

The pulp chamber extends incisally into three small pulp horns, *cornua pulpae*, which correspond with the three incisal mamelons. They are not as well developed as in the maxillary central incisor.

The pulp chamber has approximately the same shape as the external crown morphology.

The root canal is mostly oval in cross-section and flattened considerably on the mesial and distal sides. In examples with a very flat root, the root canal is often nearly divided into two canals, but in nearly all cases, the root canal constricts again at the apex to end as a single apical foramen.

Completion of *foramen apicale*: 10 years.

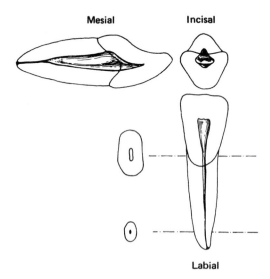

Mesial   **Incisal**

Labial

Fig. 81. Mandibular first permanent incisor.

Maxillary second permanent incisor

This tooth resembles the maxillary first permanent incisor, and the pulp cavity is accordingly similar, but is proportionately narrower because of the smaller size of the maxillary second incisor. The root canal flares out from a narrow apical foramen until it joins the fan-shaped pulp cavity, when viewed from the labial aspect. From the mesial or distal aspect, the pulp cavity is wedge-shaped. The roof of the pulp chamber has two pulp horns extending towards the mesioincisal and distoincisal angles of the crown. The outline of the pulp chamber is almost circular in cross-section compared with that of the maxillary central incisor in which it is flattened labiopalatally to an oval shape.

The root canal resembles that of the maxillary central incisor, and tapers gradually to the apical foramen where it is circular in cross-section. A constriction is also present at the level just apical to the cemento-enamel junction.

Completion of *foramen apicale*: 11 years.

110

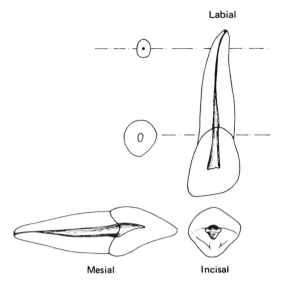

Fig. 82. Maxillary second permanent incisor.

Mandibular second permanent incisor

The general form of the pulp cavity of this tooth is similar to that of the mandibular first permanent incisor, with a simple root canal becoming gradually wider as it reaches incisally to end in a chisel-shaped pulp chamber surmounted by three small pulp horns. The only difference is that the total length of the pulp cavity is slightly longer than in the mandibular first permanent incisor.

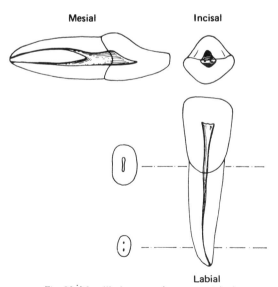

Fig. 83. Mandibular second permanent incisor.

The mesiodistal flattening of the root sometimes results in a partial division of the root canal so that two apical foramina are present at the root apex: one labial and one lingual. This is important to remember in the clinical situation, because both foramina have to be sealed off for a successful endodontic treatment. If it is assumed that only one is present, then only one will be filled and the treatment will be unsuccessful. X-ray photos are often misleading since the rays are projected labiolingually, which superimposes one canal on the other giving an image of a single canal.

The canal is mostly straight and simple, with a slight distal curvature.

Completion of *foramen apicale*: 11 years.

Maxillary permanent canine

The maxillary permanent canine has the longest root canal of all the teeth in the human dentition. It is oval in cross-section and flattened on the mesial and distal surfaces. The widest point of the root canal is at the level of the cemento-enamel junction in a labiopalatal section, from which it tapers to the single pulp horn associated with the pointed cusp of the crown. The cross-section of the root canal is circular at the apex, ending in a slightly larger apical foramen than in the maxillary incisors.

The pulp chamber itself is similar to those of the maxillary incisors, but conforming more to the pointed crown form, with one pulp horn. The pulp chamber is widest labiopalatally. It displays a slight constriction at the level just apical to the cemento-enamel junction, but to a much lesser degree than is present in the maxillary permanent incisors.

Completion of *foramen apicale*: 15 years.

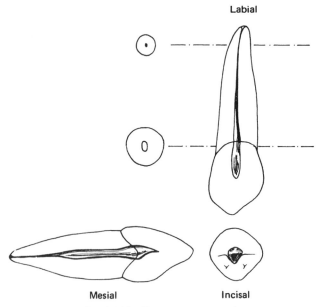

Fig. 84. Maxillary permanent canine.

Mandibular permanent canine

The pulp cavity of this tooth is best compared with that of the maxillary permanent canine. The pulp chamber extends to a point towards the cusp tip, and has the appearance of a pointed teaspoon with the hollow side facing lingually. There is one pulp horn.

The widest part of the pulp cavity lies at a point approximately level with the cemento-enamel junction. At this point, the cross-section of the root canal is oval, being flattened on its mesial and distal sides. It becomes gradually more circular towards the root apex where it tapers to the apical foramen.

An unusual variation sometimes occurs in this tooth, and which is never found in the maxillary canine: there may be a partial division of the root canal in the apical third of the root, resulting in a labial and a lingual root canal. The same problems can therefore arise with endodontic treatment as previously discussed in the description of the mandibular second permanent incisor.

Completion of *foramen apicale*: 15 years.

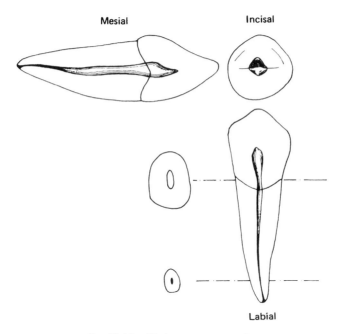

Mesial   Incisal

Labial

Fig. 85. Mandibular permanent canine.

Maxillary first premolar

This tooth has a flattened pulp cavity and is widest buccopalatally. Two pulp horns extend from the roof of the pulp chamber, one to each cusp. The buccal pulp horn is the higher.

The floor of the pulp chamber is convex with its highest point in the centre where the pulp chamber divides into two root canals. This point is approximately 2 mm apical from the level of the cemento-enamel junction. From here, the root canals narrow gradually, tapering to the root apices.

A further division may occur in cases where the buccal root is partially divided into a mesial and distal root, with corresponding mesial and distal root canals. This may also occur if the buccal root is not partially divided, but simply flattened buccopalatally, in which case there may be one or two apical foramina.

Another variation of the maxillary first premolar is a single root, flattened on its mesial and distal surfaces. In this case, there are usually two root canals, one buccal and one palatal, and these often converge to a common apical foramen. Each canal, in nearly every case, is circular in cross-section.

Completion of *foramina apicorum*: 15 years.

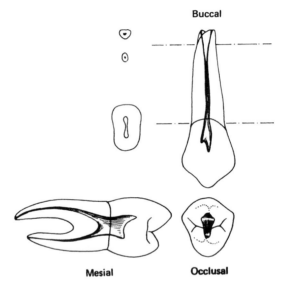

Buccal

Mesial　　　　**Occlusal**

Fig. 86. Maxillary first premolar.

Mandibular first premolar

The pulp chamber of this tooth is widest buccolingually. It has two pulp horns, one buccal and one lingual, of which the buccal is considerably higher, with the result that the roof of the pulp chamber tilts lingually, at approximately 45°, parallel with the occlusal surface. This is important to remember during cavity preparations, so that the drill is also inclined lingually to avoid exposing the buccal pulp horn.

The floor of the pulp chamber is positioned 2 or 3 mm apical to the level of the cemento-enamel junction, where it narrows down to join the root canal, which at this point is oval-shaped, and flattened on the mesial and distal sides. This root canal usually extends uninterrupted to the root apex, but may occasionally divide into a buccal and a lingual canal halfway, before joining up again in the apical third of the root, to exit at a common single apical foramen.

The apical third of the canal tends to curve distally.

Completion of *foramen apicale*: 15 years.

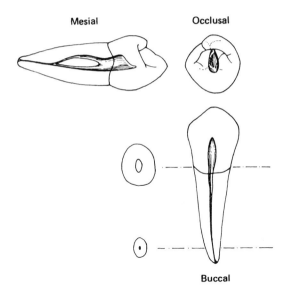

Mesial

Occlusal

Buccal

Fig. 87. Mandibular first premolar.

Maxillary second premolar

The pulp chamber of the maxillary second premolar is oval in cross-section and flattened on the mesial and distal sides. There are two pulp horns, one to each cusp, and the buccal pulp horn is higher than the palatal pulp horn. The base of the pulp

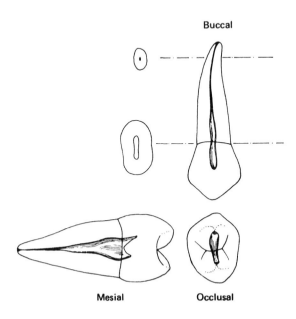

Buccal

Mesial

Occlusal

Fig. 88. Maxillary second premolar.

chamber is placed further apically than that of the maxillary first premolar, before narrowing into a single root canal, which tapers gradually to the root apex. This canal is considerably flattened on its mesial and distal sides, and has an elongated oval cross-section. This becomes more circular in the region of the root apex.

Very occasionally, the maxillary second premolar has two roots, or a partial division of its root in the apical third. When this occurs, the root canal also divides to end in two apical foramina in the same way as in maxillary first premolar.

The root canal sometimes divides into a buccal and a palatal component when a single root is present, but they rejoin in the apical third of the root, and end at a somewhat larger, elongated apical foramen.

Pulp exposures during cavity preparations occur just as easily in this tooth as in the mandibular first premolar. This is also due to the fact that both pulp horns, especially the buccal, extend deep into the cusps. The cusps are of equal height, but the pulp horns are not, with the result that the buccal pulp horn is the most frequently involved in the event of an iatrogenic pulp exposure.

Completion of *foramen apicale*: 15 years.

Mandibular second premolar

This tooth has a flat pulp chamber, its greatest dimension being buccolingual. It has two pulp horns and a single root canal. There is a considerable difference in height between the two pulp horns, of several millimetres, the buccal being the larger of the two, although not as markedly as in the mandibular first premolar. Because of this, and the shallower lingual inclination of the occlusal surface, accidental pulp exposures occur less frequently in this tooth as in the mandibular first premolar.

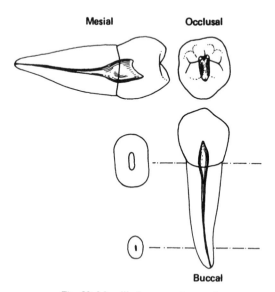

Fig. 89. Mandibular second premolar.

Many of the three-cusped versions of this tooth have three pulp horns, although the usual number quoted is two, and in all cases, the lingual pulp horn is better developed than that of the mandibular first premolar.

The root canal is oval in cross-section, becoming more circular towards the apex. It can vary in the same way as that of the mandibular first premolar.

Completion of *foramen apicale*: 15 years.

Maxillary first permanent molar

The pulp chamber of the maxillary first permanent molar is approximately square in cross-section with concave walls. There are four pulp horns, one to each cusp, of which the mesiobuccal is the highest. Both mesial pulp horns are higher than the distal pulp horns, and the distopalatal is the smallest of them all.

At the level approximately 1 mm apical to the cemento-enamel junction, the square cross-section of the pulp chamber gradually changes to a triangular shape, with the three corners corresponding with the three funnel-shaped entrances of the three separate root canals.

The root canals are proportionate in size to the three roots, so that the palatal canal is the longest and widest, whilst the mesiobuccal canal is narrower and

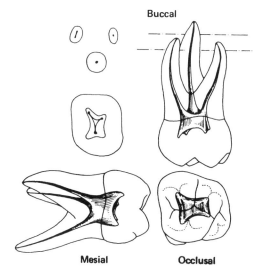

Fig. 90. Maxillary first permanent molar.

somewhat flattened with a marked distal curvature. The distobuccal canal is more circular in cross-section, narrow and also curves distally. It is the shortest of the three canals.

The flattening of the mesiobuccal root canal sometimes results in its being partially divided into two branches, one buccal and one palatal, but these usually rejoin at the root apex at a single apical foramen. This variation is difficult to detect radiographically, and can give complications during an endodontic treatment.

In the event of the rare presence of the variation, *radix paramolaris*, the maxillary first permanent molar will also have an extra root canal in this accessory rootlet.

Completion of *foramina apicorum*: 10 years.

Mandibular first permanent molar

The pulp chamber of the mandibular first permanent molar is wider buccolingually at its mesial end than at the distal end. It has a pulp horn under each cusp viz. three buccal and two lingual, and in decreasing order of height, these are as follows: mesiobuccal, mesiolingual, distobuccal, distolingual, distal.

In cross-section, the outline of the pulp chamber is roughly triangular in shape with rounded corners, and elongated mesiodistally. Each corner of the triangle is situated above the entrance of a root canal. The floor of the pulp chamber is convex, and the entrances to the root canals are funnel-shaped.

The mesial root has two root canals: one buccal and one lingual, but in some younger specimens they may be fused together as a single ribbon-like canal, compressed on its mesial and distal sides.

The shape of the apical foramen in the mesial root is determined by the level at which the two root canals join. This usually takes place a few millimetres before the root apex is reached, resulting in a single, circular or oval-shaped apical foramen. If, however, the two root canals fuse at the level of the root apex itself, then the result is an apical split or even two separate foramina which may or may not be joined by an extremely fine split extending between them.

The single root canal in the distal root is rounder in cross-section, relatively wide, and less curved than the two mesial root canals.

An extra root canal is present in the rare variation of *radix entomolaris*, a lingually positioned, accessory rootlet.

Completion of *foramina apicorum*: 10 years.

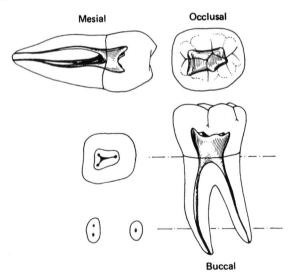

Fig. 91. Mandibular first permanent molar.

Maxillary second permanent molar

The pulp cavity of this tooth has approximately the same shape as that of the maxillary first permanent molar except that it is slightly smaller overall. The root canals are also less divergent.

The pulp chamber is mesiodistally compressed so that it is widest buccopalatally, like the crown. The roof of the pulp chamber extends occlusally to four distinct pulp horns, each directed to one of the four cusps. The two mesial pulp horns are the largest, and the distopalatal is the smallest, to the extent that it is hardly discernible in specimens with a considerably reduced distopalatal cusp. The three pulp horns of the other three cusps, which comprise the occlusal trigon, are always present, however.

The floor of the pulp chamber is triangular, with a funnel-shaped root canal entrance to each corner. Normally speaking, this tooth has three single root canals, but very occasionally an extra canal may be present if the mesiobuccal root is very wide and the canal within it bifurcates. Another possible but rare variation is an extra root canal within an accessory root, the *radix paramolaris*.

The size and shape of the root canals are determined by the shapes of the roots. In the case of partial fusion of the roots, the root canals remain almost always individual.

Completion of *foramina apicorum*: 16–17 years.

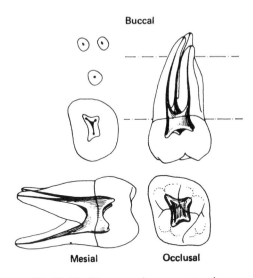

Buccal

Mesial   **Occlusal**

Fig. 92. Maxillary second permanent molar.

Mandibular second permanent molar

The shape of the pulp cavity of this tooth bears a general resemblance to that of the mandibular first permanent molar with the exception that it is shorter mesiodistally, with four pulp horns instead of five. The pulp chamber has a mesiodistally elongated triangular shape with rounded corners in occlusal cross-section, and is widest buccolingually at its mesial end. The three funnel-shaped root canal entrances are situated at the corners.

There are three root canals. The mesiolingual and mesiobuccal canals are situated next to each other in the mesial root, and a larger, single canal with an oval cross-section is situated in the distal root.

The variation, *radix entomolaris*, is responsible for a fourth, lingually placed canal in the rare event of this accessory rootlet being present, in which case the root canal entrance is situated on the lingual side of the distal root canal entrance.

In young specimens of the mandibular second permanent molar, in which the roots are not fully developed, the mesial root has a single, ribbon-like canal with a figure-of-eight cross-section. This becomes divided in time with further deposition of dentine. A consequence of this development is that the mesial root apex may have a single, double or split-shaped apical foramen.

Completion of *foramina apicorum*: 16–17 years.

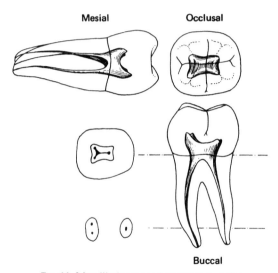

Fig. 93. Mandibular second permanent molar.

Maxillary third molar

A detailed description of a typical third molar pulp morphology is of little use since this tooth displays so many different morphological variations. All the author can offer here is a few general comments about its pulp anatomy, and the advice to study any diagnostic X-ray photos very carefully should this tooth be of clinical endodontic importance.

Usually all three of the cusps that make up the trigon are present in the maxillary third molar, and one can reasonably assume that three pulp horns will be present, each corresponding to one of the cusps. Of these the mesiobuccal is usually the highest.

The root morphology and the corresponding endodontic anatomy of the maxillary third molar are impossible to guess, in the clinical situation, by looking at the crown, and X-ray photos are always to be advised.

In the case of peg-shaped third molars, there is a single root canal which is circular in cross-section. If the third molar resembles the maxillary second molar, then there is a chance that the root and pulp morphology is similar. In most cases, however, the roots of the maxillary third molar are to a greater or lesser degree fused together, and may form a single, irregular, funnel-shaped root canal.

Completion of *foramina apicorum*: 21 years.

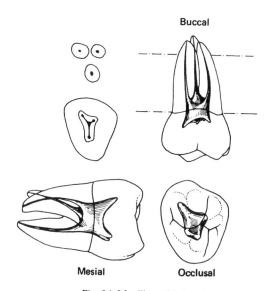

Buccal

Mesial **Occlusal**

Fig. 94. Maxillary third molar.

Mandibular third molar

A reasonably 'normal' specimen of this tooth resembles the exterior as well as the interior of the mandibular second permanent molar, but differs in having shorter root canals with a more pronounced distal curvature. The 'normal' form presents, however, just as frequently as the other variations in form, which makes it difficult to describe a typical mandibular third molar pulp morphology.

As a rule, it may be assumed that there are the same number of pulp horns as there are cusps, but unfortunately, this endodontic guesswork does not extend to the root canals, so that X-ray photos are, once again, imperative in the clinical situation.

The root canals are usually wider than those of the other mandibular molars, and end in rather large apical foramina. A common variation is the mandibular third molar with a single fused root mass containing a very wide conical root canal ending in a distally-curved root apex.

Completion of *foramina apicorum*: 21 years.

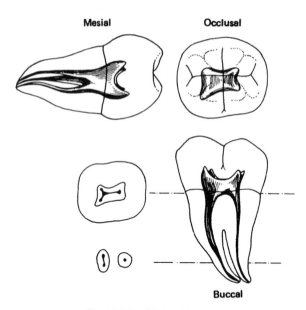

Mesial

Occlusal

Buccal

Fig. 95. Mandibular third molar.

Section 4

Appendix

Tables

Table 1, 'Chronology of the Deciduous Dentition', and *Table* 3, 'Chronology of the Permanent Dentition' are based on the work of Logan and Krönfeld (slightly modified by Schour). They are only a guide, for if a tooth erupts up to two years before or after the dates given, this is still considered to be normal. As a rule, clinical investigations are usually made if the eruption date extends beyond these limits.

The dimensions given in *Tables* 2 and 3 are based on the work of Black.

Table 1. **Chronology of the deciduous dentition**

Tooth	Initial calcification	Completion of crown	Eruption	Completion of roots
Maxillary first incisor	3–4 months in utero	4 months	$7\frac{1}{2}$ months	$1\frac{1}{2}$–2 years
Mandibular first incisor	$4\frac{1}{2}$ months in utero	4 months	$6\frac{1}{2}$ months	$1\frac{1}{2}$–2 years
Maxillary second incisor	$4\frac{1}{2}$ months in utero	5 months	8 months	$1\frac{1}{2}$–2 years
Mandibular second incisor	$4\frac{1}{2}$ months in utero	$4\frac{1}{2}$ months	7 months	$1\frac{1}{2}$–2 years
Maxillary canine	5 months in utero	9 months	16–20 months	$2\frac{1}{2}$–3 years
Mandibular canine	5 months in utero	9 months	16–20 months	$2\frac{1}{2}$–3 years
Maxillary first molar	5 months in utero	6 months	12–16 months	2–$2\frac{1}{4}$ years
Mandibular first molar	5 months in utero	6 months	12–16 months	2–$2\frac{1}{2}$ years
Maxillary second molar	6 months in utero	10–12 months	$1\frac{3}{4}$–$2\frac{1}{2}$ years	3 years
Mandibular second molar	6 months in utero	10–12 months	$1\frac{3}{4}$–$2\frac{1}{2}$ years	3 years

Order of Eruption of the Deciduous Teeth
1. Mandibular central incisors
2. Maxillary central incisors
3. Mandibular lateral incisors
4. Maxillary lateral incisors
5. First molars
6. Canines
7. Second molars

Order of Eruption of Maxillary Deciduous Teeth
A   B   D   C   E

Order of Eruption of Mandibular Deciduous Teeth
A   B   D   C   E

Table 2. Average dimensions of the deciduous teeth

Tooth	Mesiodistal width (mm)	Labiolingual width (mm)	Length of crown (mm)	Length of root (mm)	Total length (mm)
Maxillary first incisor	6·5	5·0	6·0	10·0	16·0
Maxillary second incisor	5·2	4·0	5·6	10·2	15·8
Maxillary canine	6·8	7·0	6·5	13·0	19·5
Maxillary first molar	7·1	8·5	5·1	10·0	15·1
Maxillary second molar	8·4	10·0	5·7	11·7	17·4
Mandibular first incisor	4·0	4·0	5·0	9·0	14·0
Mandibular second incisor	4·5	4·0	5·2	9·8	15·0
Mandibular canine	5·5	4·9	6·0	11·2	17·2
Mandibular first molar	7·7	7·0	6·0	9·8	15·8
Mandibular second molar	9·7	8·7	5·5	12·5	18·0

Table 3. Chronology of the permanent dentition

Tooth	Initial calcification	Completion of crown	Eruption	Completion of crown
Maxillary first incisor	3–4 months	4–5 years	7–8 years	10 years
Mandibular first incisor	3–4 months	4–5 years	6–7 years	9 years
Maxillary second incisor	10–12 months	4–5 years	8–9 years	11 years
Mandibular second incisor	3–4 months	4–5 years	7–8 years	10 years
Maxillary canine	4–5 months	6–7 years	11–12 years	13–15 years
Mandibular canine	4–5 months	6–7 years	9–10 years	12–14 years
Maxillary first premolar	$1\frac{1}{2}$–18 years	5–6 years	10–11 years	12–13 years
Mandibular first premolar	$1\frac{3}{4}$–2 years	5–6 years	10–12 years	12–13 years
Maxillary second premolar	2–$2\frac{1}{2}$ years	6–7 years	10–12 years	12–14 years
Mandibular second premolar	$2\frac{1}{4}$–$2\frac{1}{2}$ years	6–7 years	11–12 years	13–14 years
Maxillary first molar	Birth or slightly before	$2\frac{1}{2}$–3 years	6–7 years	9–10 years
Mandibular first molar	Birth or slightly before	$2\frac{1}{2}$–3 years	6–7 years	9–10 years
Maxillary second molar	$2\frac{1}{2}$–3 years	7–8 years	12–13 years	14–16 years
Mandibular second molar	$2\frac{1}{2}$–3 years	7–8 years	12–13 years	14–15 years
Maxillary third molar	7–9 years	12–16 years	17–21 years	18–25 years
Mandibular third molar	8–10 years	12–16 years	17–21 years	18–25 years

Table 4. Average dimensions of the permanent teeth

Tooth	Mesiodistal width (mm)	Labiolingual width (mm)	Length of crown (mm)	Length of root (mm)	Total length (mm)
Maxillary first incisor	8·5	7·0	10·5	13·0	23·5
Maxillary second incisor	6·5	6·0	9·0	13·0	22·0
Maxillary canine	7·5	8·0	10·0	17·0	27·0
Maxillary first premolar	7·0	9·0	8·5	14·5	23·0
Maxillary second premolar	7·0	9·0	8·5	14·0	22·5
Maxillary first molar	10·5	11·0	7·5	12·5	20·0
Maxillary second molar	9·5	11·0	7·0	11·5	18·5
Maxillary third molar	8·5	10·0	6·5	11·0	17·5
Mandibular first incisor	5·0	6·0	9·0	12·5	21·5
Mandibular second incisor	5·5	6·5	9·5	14·0	23·5
Mandibular canine	7·0	7·5	11·0	15·5	26·5
Mandibular first premolar	7·0	7·5	8·5	14·0	22·5
Mandibular second premolar	7·0	8·0	8·0	14·5	22·5
Mandibular first molar	11·0	10·0	7·5	14·0	21·5
Mandibular second molar	10·5	10·0	7·0	12·0	19·0
Mandibular third molar	10·0	9·5	7·0	11·0	18·0

Order of Eruption of the Permanent Teeth
1. First molars
2. Mandibular first and second incisors
3. Maxillary first incisors
4. Maxillary second incisors
5. Mandibular canines
6. First premolars
7. Second premolars
8. Maxillary canines
9. Second molars
10. Third molars

Order of Eruption of Maxillary Permanent Teeth
6 1 2 4 5 3 7 8

Order of Eruption of Mandibular Permanent Teeth
6 1 2 3 4 5 7 8

Glossary

Alveolar crest	The highest part of the alveolar process.
Alveolar process	The bone of the maxilla and the mandible which surrounds and supports the teeth.
Apex	The tip of the root.
Attrition	Wearing down of the occlusal surfaces by use.
Bicuspid	*See* Premolar
Bifurcation	Division of the root into two parts.
Buccal	The outer surface of posterior teeth in contact with the cheek.
Canine	The tooth third from the midline used for gripping and tearing food.
Canine eminence	The bulge on the labial aspect of the maxilla caused by the large roots of the canine teeth.
Carabelli, cusp of	An extra cusp on the mesiolingual cusp of the upper first permanent molar in 50–75 per cent of cases.
Carnivore	An animal with teeth adapted for meat eating.
Cemento-enamel junction	The line formed by the division between the enamel of the crown and the cementum of the root. Cervical margin or line.
Cementum	The layer of calcified tissue covering the root of the tooth.
Cervical	Describes the area near the cemento-enamel junction.
Cervical line/margin	The line formed by the cemento-enamel junction.
Cervix	The narrow part of the tooth where the root and the crown are joined. Cervical margin/line/cemento-enamel junction.
Cheek teeth	The posterior teeth, i.e. premolars and molars.
Cingulum	Rounded protuberance on cervical third of crown.
Cornu	A projection of the pulp, also called a horn.
Crown, anatomical	The enamel-covered part of the tooth.
Crown, clinical	The part of the crown that appears above the gingiva.
Cusp	A peak on the occlusal surface of a tooth.
Cuspid	*See* Canine.
Deciduous	Describes the primary dentition.
Dentine	The body of the tooth, underneath the enamel and cementum, formed by odontoblast cells.
Developmental groove/fissure	Groove dividing the cusps.
Distal	That part of a tooth farthest away from the midline.
Embrasure	The space formed where teeth diverge from contact points.
Enamel	Hard vitreous tissue covering the crown of the tooth formed by ameloblast cells.

Eruption	The process by which a tooth appears through the bone and the gingiva.
Exfoliation	The shedding of the primary teeth.
Fissure	A developmental cleft, usually found on the occlusal or buccal surface.
Gingiva	The gum surrounding the tooth.
Incisal edge	The biting edge of anterior teeth.
Incisor	The teeth first and second from the midline used for cutting food.
Labial	The outer surface of anterior teeth in contact with the lips.
Lingual	The inner surface of a tooth in contact with the tongue.
Mamelon	Small protuberances, usually three in number, present on the incisal edge of a newly-erupted incisor.
Mandible	The lower jaw.
Marginal ridge	Ridges of enamel at the mesial and distal edges of a tooth.
Maxilla	The upper jaw.
Maxillary sinus/antrum	An air space within the maxilla connected to the the nasal cavity.
Median plane	The bisecting line of the body.
Median/midline	The vertical bisecting line of the jaw.
Mesial	The proximal surface of a tooth nearer the midline
Molar	The teeth sixth, seventh and eighth from the midline in the permanent dentition, and fourth and fifth in the deciduous dentition, used for grinding food.
Oblique ridge	The triangular ridge of enamel running obliquely across the occlusal surface of maxillary molars.
Occlusal	The biting surface.
Occlusion	The relation of upper and lower teeth when the jaws are closed, although there are many definitions from which to choose!
Palatal	The inner surface of the upper teeth in contact with the palate. The term 'lingual' may also be used.
Palate	The roof of the mouth.
Pit	Small, deep depression in the enamel of a tooth.
Premolar	The teeth fourth and fifth from the midline used both for gripping and grinding food. Also called bicuspid.
Proximal	The surface of a tooth in contact with its neighbour. May refer to mesial or distal surface.
Pulp	The vital part of a tooth containing the nerves and blood supply.

Pulp chamber	The cavity within the crown containing the pulp; the root canals are confluent with it.
Resorption	The process by which the root tissue of the deciduous tooth is absorbed back into its developing successor.
Ridge	Narrow, elongated protrusion on the surface of a tooth.
Root	The cementum-covered part of the tooth which is embedded in the bone, and which supports the tooth.
Root canal	A funnel-shaped passage inside the root containing part of the pulp.
Root trunk	The part of the root between the cervix and the point of separation of the roots.
Trigon	A triangular group of cusps: mesiobuccal, distobuccal, and mesiopalatal which enclose the central fossa, characteristic to all maxillary molars.
Tubercle	A rounded projection on the surface of the crown, often a deviation from normal form.

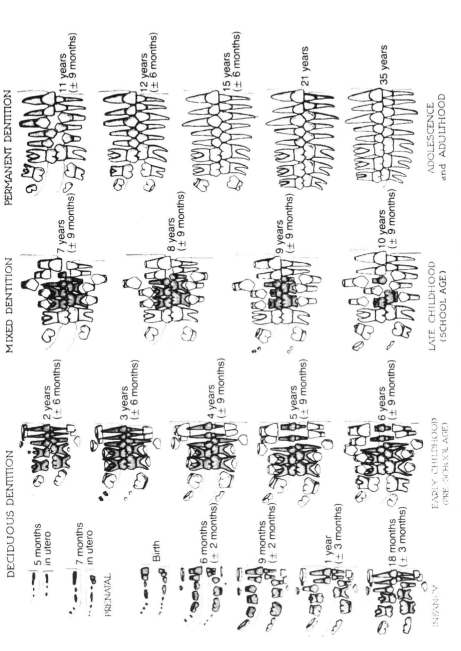

Fig. 96. Development of the human dentition.

131

Bibliography

Anderson D. J. and Buxton R. (1981) *Pocket Etymology of Medical Terms*. Bristol, Bristol Classical Press.

Andlaw R. J. and Rock W. P. (1982) *A Manual of Paedodontics*. Edinburgh, Churchill Livingstone.

Berkovitz B. K. B., Holland G. R. and Moxham B. J. (1977) *A Colour Atlas and Textbook of Oral Anatomy*. London, Wolfe Medical.

Berkovitz B. K. B. and Moxham B. J. (1977) *Multiple Choice Questions in the Anatomical Sciences for Students of Dentistry*. Bristol, Wright.

Kraus B. S., Jordan R. E. and Abrams L. (1969) *Dental Anatomy and Occlusion*. Baltimore, Williams & Wilkins.

Scott J. H. and Symons N. B. B. (1981) *Introduction to Dental Anatomy*. Edinburgh, Churchill Livingstone.

Wheeler R. C. (1962) *An Atlas of Tooth Form*. London, Saunders.

Wheeler R. C. (1974) *A Textbook of Dental Anatomy and Physiology*. Philadelphia, Saunders.

Index

134